Molecular Docking - Recent Advances

Edited by Erman Salih Istifli

Published in London, United Kingdom

Molecular Docking - Recent Advances
http://dx.doi.org/10.5772/intechopen.100665
Edited by Erman Salih Istifli

Contributors
Mauricio Carrillo-Tripp, Aldo Herrera-Rodulfo, Mariana Andrade-Medina, Erman Salih Istifli, Iqbal Azad, Saliha Ece Acuner, Selin Sezer, Sefika Feyza Maden, Kishor Danao, Deweshri Nandurkar, Vijayshri Rokde, Ruchi Shivhare, Ujwala Mahajan, Rupesh Chikhale, Mohit Umare, Fai A. Alkathiri, Elena Kalinichenko, Aliaksandr Faryna

First published in London, United Kingdom, 2023 by IntechOpen
IntechOpen is the global imprint of INTECHOPEN LIMITED, registered in England and Wales, registration number: 11086078, 5 Princes Gate Court, London, SW7 2QJ, United Kingdom

British Library Cataloguing-in-Publication Data
A catalogue record for this book is available from the British Library

Additional hard and PDF copies can be obtained from orders@intechopen.com

Molecular Docking - Recent Advances
Edited by Erman Salih Istifli
p. cm.

This title is part of the Biomedical Engineering Book Series, Volume 15
Topic: Bioinformatics and Medical Informatics
Series Editor: Robert Koprowski
Topic Editor: Slawomir Wilczynski

Print ISBN 978-1-80356-467-8
Online ISBN 978-1-80356-468-5
eBook (PDF) ISBN 978-1-80356-469-2
ISSN 2631-5343

IntechOpen Book Series

Biomedical Engineering

Volume 15

Aims and Scope of the Series

Biomedical Engineering is one of the fastest-growing interdisciplinary branches of science and industry. The combination of electronics and computer science with biology and medicine has improved patient diagnosis, reduced rehabilitation time, and helped to facilitate a better quality of life. Nowadays, all medical imaging devices, medical instruments, or new laboratory techniques result from the cooperation of specialists in various fields. The series of Biomedical Engineering books covers such areas of knowledge as chemistry, physics, electronics, medicine, and biology. This series is intended for doctors, engineers, and scientists involved in biomedical engineering or those wanting to start working in this field.

Meet the Series Editor

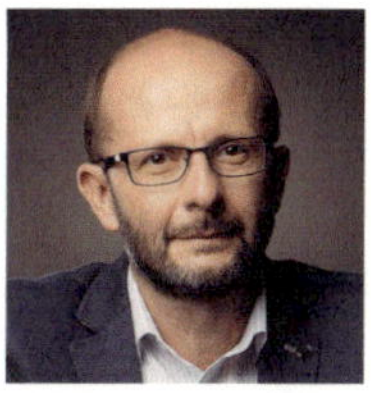

Robert Koprowski, MD (1997), Ph.D. (2003), Habilitation (2015), is an employee of the University of Silesia, Poland, Institute of Computer Science, Department of Biomedical Computer Systems. For 20 years, he has studied the analysis and processing of biomedical images, emphasizing the full automation of measurement for a large inter-individual variability of patients. Dr. Koprowski has authored more than a hundred research papers with dozens in impact factor (IF) journals and has authored or co-authored six books. Additionally, he is the author of several national and international patents in the field of biomedical devices and imaging. Since 2011, he has been a reviewer of grants and projects (including EU projects) in biomedical engineering.

Meet the Volume Editor

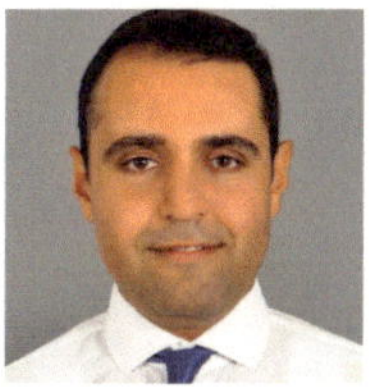

Dr. Erman Salih Istifli's postdoctoral studies include the discovery of candidate phytochemicals in the treatment of SARS-CoV-2, DNA–ligand interactions, and the discovery of plant-based natural inhibitors against certain enzymes (AChE, BChE, alpha-amylase, alpha-glucosidase, and tyrosinase) that are important regulators of human health. He has been the scientific editor of the *International Journal of Plant Based Pharmaceuticals* since 2021.

Contents

Preface

Molecular docking, the first algorithms of which were written in the 1980s, has now become a routine computational method in the discovery of effective molecules (high-throughput screening, drug repurposing) for curable and even incurable diseases. It is used to elucidate receptor–ligand intermolecular interactions at the atom level and to predict the possible binding conformations of molecular complexes (DNA–protein, RNA–protein, protein-protein, or protein-small molecule) whose crystal structure is still unknown. Although these are among the routine uses of molecular docking, from a reductionist scientific point of view, the capacity of this technique to illuminate different molecular phenomena is limited only by imagination, and its use in biology and medicine is diversifying day by day.

With the outbreak of the COVID-19 pandemic worldwide, it became clear how this technique, which made a very rapid entry into the biological sciences in the last decade, has contributed greatly to new drug discovery and drug development. It has also made a significant contribution to the identification of new molecular targets related to COVID-19 treatment. In addition, multiple human protein targets were determined in the treatment of COVID-19 via the molecular docking technique, which led to the adoption of the 'multi-target' approach in drug screening studies. Strikingly, although molecular docking is used quite frequently in hit identification and lead optimization, it has also begun to be used in bioremediation for predicting pollutants that can be degraded by different enzymes.

Despite molecular docking being a promising technique in biology, biochemistry, and medicine, the conformation of the obtained molecular complexes and the compatibility of the binding energies with the experimental data is still debatable and, thus, more refinement of scoring functions is required. Hopefully, with the development of new docking algorithms and approaches (e.g., flexible docking, solvated docking, covalent docking, and consensus docking), the prediction of molecular complexes in accordance with experimental data can now be made more accurately. In addition, the contribution of molecular dynamics simulations and free energy calculations in refining the molecular docking binding energy is invaluable and cannot be ignored.

This book presents current studies on computational molecular docking as well as discusses the fundamentals of the technique. It is designed for researchers of all levels.

Dr. Erman Salih Istifli
Biology, Faculty of Science and Literature,
Cukurova University,
Adana, Turkey

Section 1

Introduction

Chapter 1

Introductory Chapter: Molecular Docking – The Transition from the Micro Nature of Small Molecules to the Macro World

Erman Salih Istifli

1. Introduction

Molecular docking is a frequently employed bioinformatics method that is capable of predicting with great accuracy (when the initial structure preparation is done properly) the conformation of small molecular weight ligands (Latin *ligandus*, gerundive of *ligare* "to bind") within the binding sites of proteins, enzymes, RNA or DNA macromolecular targets [1–5]. Since the development of its first algorithm in the 1980s, molecular docking has been an indispensable tool in drug discovery, however, following the further recognition of its ability to highly predict intermolecular interactions by researchers, it has also found widespread use in biochemistry, medicinal chemistry, pharmacy, microbiology, genetics, advanced biophysics, and even the textile industry. Although it is not the specific subject of this introductory chapter, the main principle of molecular docking, as software, is based on two main processes: a. *conformational search*, and, b. determination of the *binding energetics*. In the conformational search step, the most likely conformation (minimum energy solution) of the ligand on the target receptor is identified by modifying its structural parameters, such as torsional, translational, and rotational degrees of freedom. In the calculation step of the binding energy of the ligand-receptor complex, which is predicted by conformational search, a binding constant (K_d or K_i) and *Gibbs free energy* value ($\Delta G°$=kcal/mol) are produced using different scoring functions [1, 6–11].

2. What advantages did molecular docking technique offer us?

In the last two decades, molecular docking has found significant use in the discipline of molecular biology in addition to structure-based drug design (SBDD). For instance, while the molecular docking method predicts the interactions between enzymes and their substrates, quite accurately in terms of binding free energy and conformation [12–15], it has also proven its ability to calculate the negative functional effects of induced mutations in proteins as well as the effects of naturally occurring point mutations on enzyme-substrate binding [16–19]. Thus, molecular docking offers a powerful option for investigating the correlation between structure and function. While the utilization of molecular docking in biochemistry is generally

IntechOpen

aimed at confirming data related to enzyme inhibitory activity, such as experimental dissociation constant (K_d) or half-maximal inhibitory concentration (IC_{50}) [20–24], in microbiology, it is widely used to theoretically verify the minimum inhibitory concentration (MIC) values of natural herbal extracts or synthetic components targeted against bacterial enzymes [25–29]. Recently, although molecular docking programs have not been specifically designed to characterize ligand-DNA interactions, the molecular docking method has now been frequently used to predict the binding modes and affinity of small molecules on DNA, especially in genotoxicity studies [30–35]. Last but not least, the inherent nature of molecular docking, which is based on biochemistry and biophysics, has allowed it to take place even in the COVID-19 pandemic, which has severely affected the world agenda, societies, and the global economy for about 2 years. This method has ultimately become a principle component in bioinformatics-based drug-discovery campaigns against the SARS-CoV-2 virus [36–41].

3. Molecular docking is in principle closely connected with molecular dynamics simulations

As commonly known, intracellular receptor-ligand interactions are dynamic phenomena by nature, where ions and water molecules in this milieu have undeniable importance during these intermolecular reactions. At the same time, the inherent flexibility of the interacting protein partners and ligands is an important variable that has to be taken into account in docking calculations. Therefore, considering these variables, molecular docking techniques have evolved further over time and new docking algorithms (ex. flexible receptor-flexible ligand docking or solvated docking) have been developed to produce more accurate receptor-ligand poses [42–45]. However, simulating the movements of all types of atoms around the reaction site is still beyond the limits of the molecular docking technique. In this context, the molecular dynamics simulations have proved to be indispensable molecular interaction simulation methods used as a complement to the molecular docking technique in order to study the receptor-ligand binding dynamics and the time-dependent evolution of the resulting complex. Therefore, the molecular docking technique should be supported by molecular dynamics simulations, regardless of which biological problem it is used to solve.

4. Conclusion

A feature of biological macromolecules or synthetic chemical compounds is that the basic building blocks come together to form larger building blocks, which then come together to form even larger structures, and the process continues in the same way. The structure and function of these macromolecules composed of small monomers are frequently quite different from the building blocks that compose them, and such phenomena are referred as '*emergence*' if you ask physicists or biologists. Consequently, it is almost impossible to explain the basis of the *emergence* phenomenon using scientific reductionism. However, molecular docking, which is one of the most powerful supportive tools of scientific reductionism today, can now display atomic interactions (with almost all the details) in intermolecular reactions on a computer screen, which was almost impossible until about 45–50 years ago. Furthermore, with the ever-developing disciplines such as genomics, molecular biology, biochemistry, and genetics, molecular docking has become a more powerful tool today and the scientific disciplines it can directly contribute to are increasing at the same rate. Thus, the importance of scientific reductionism, therefore molecular docking, in imagining the '*big biological window*' seems likely to continue with increasing importance. In summary, this book is an ultimate reference guide for researchers working in the fields of experimental biology and bioinformatics who would like to understand the principles of the molecular docking technique and integrate it into their research areas, as well as students who are prospective in increasing their knowledge about molecular simulations.

Author details

Erman Salih Istifli
Department of Biology, Faculty of Science and Literature, Cukurova University, Adana, Turkey

*Address all correspondence to: esistifli@cu.edu.tr

References

[1] Ferreira LG, Dos Santos RN, Oliva G, Andricopulo AD. Molecular docking and structure-based drug design strategies. Molecules. 2015;**20**(7):13384-13421

[2] Morris GM, Lim-Wilby M. Molecular docking. In: Kukol A, editor. Molecular Modeling of Proteins. Totowa, NJ: Humana; 2008. pp. 365-382

[3] Pagadala NS, Syed K, Tuszynski J. Software for molecular docking: A review. Biophysical Reviews. 2017;**9**(2):91-102

[4] Gschwend DA, Good AC, Kuntz ID. Molecular docking towards drug discovery. Journal of Molecular Recognition: An Interdisciplinary Journal. 1996;**9**(2):175-186

[5] Fan J, Fu A, Zhang L. Progress in molecular docking. Quantitative Biology. 2019;**7**(2):83-89

[6] Dias R, de Azevedo J, Walter F. Molecular docking algorithms. Current Drug Targets. 2008;**9**(12):1040-1047

[7] Sethi A, Joshi K, Sasikala K, Alvala M. Molecular docking in modern drug discovery: Principles and recent applications. Drug discovery and Development-New Advances. 2019;**2**:1-21

[8] Halperin I, Ma B, Wolfson H, Nussinov R. Principles of docking: An overview of search algorithms and a guide to scoring functions. Proteins: Structure, Function, and Bioinformatics. 2002;**47**(4):409-443

[9] Yuriev E, Holien J, Ramsland PA. Improvements, trends, and new ideas in molecular docking: 2012-2013 in review. Journal of Molecular Recognition. 2015;**28**(10):581-604

[10] Andrusier N, Mashiach E, Nussinov R, Wolfson HJ. Principles of flexible protein–protein docking. Proteins: Structure, Function, and Bioinformatics. 2008;**73**(2):271-289

[11] Prieto-Martínez FD, Arciniega M, Medina-Franco JL. Molecular docking: Current advances and challenges. TIP. Revista especializada en ciencias químico-biológicas. 2018;**21**(Suppl. 1): 65-87

[12] Luniwal A, Wang L, Pavlovsky A, Erhardt PW, Viola RE. Molecular docking and enzymatic evaluation to identify selective inhibitors of aspartate semialdehyde dehydrogenase. Bioorganic & Medicinal Chemistry. 2012;**20**(9):2950-2956

[13] Rudnitskaya A, Török B, Török M. Molecular docking of enzyme inhibitors: A computational tool for structure-based drug design. Biochemistry and Molecular Biology Education. 2010;**38**(4):261-265

[14] Udatha DBRK, Sugaya N, Olsson L, Panagiotou G. How well do the substrates KISS the enzyme? Molecular docking program selection for feruloyl esterases. Scientific Reports. 2012;**2**(1):1-8

[15] Burmaoglu S, Kazancioglu EA, Kazancioglu MZ, Sağlamtaş R, Yalcin G, Gulcin I, et al. Synthesis, molecular docking and some metabolic enzyme inhibition properties of biphenyl-substituted chalcone derivatives. Journal of Molecular Structure. 2022;**1254**:132358

[16] Karaytuğ T, Arabacı N, İstifli ES. Microbial and bioinformatics approach in biofuel production. In: Bioenergy Research: Basic and Advanced Concepts. Singapore: Springer; 2021. pp. 257-306

[17] Yu J, Shi J, Zhang Y, Yu Z. Molecular docking and site-directed mutagenesis of dichloromethane dehalogenase to improve enzyme activity for dichloromethane degradation. Applied Biochemistry and Biotechnology. 2020;**190**(2):487-505

[18] Chiappori F, D'Ursi P, Merelli I, Milanesi L, Rovida E. In silico saturation mutagenesis and docking screening for the analysis of protein-ligand interaction: The Endothelial Protein C Receptor case study. BMC Bioinformatics. 2009;**10**(12):1-8

[19] Go MK, Zhao LN, Xue B, Supekar S, Robinson RC, Fan H, et al. Directed computational evolution of quorum-quenching lactonases from the amidohydrolase superfamily. Structure. 2020;**28**(6):635-642

[20] Deepa PR, Vandhana S, Muthukumaran S, Umashankar V, Jayanthi U, Krishnakumar S. Chemical inhibition of fatty acid synthase: Molecular docking analysis and biochemical validation in ocular cancer cells. Journal of Ocular Biology, Diseases, and Informatics. 2010;**3**(4):117-128

[21] Mathew B, Mathew GE, Uçar G, Baysal I, Suresh J, Vilapurathu JK, et al. Development of fluorinated methoxylated chalcones as selective monoamine oxidase-B inhibitors: Synthesis, biochemistry and molecular docking studies. Bioorganic Chemistry. 2015;**62**:22-29

[22] Günsel A, Yıldırım A, Taslimi P, Erden Y, Taskin-Tok T, Pişkin H, et al. Cytotoxicity effects and biochemical investigation of novel tetrakis-phthalocyanines bearing 2-thiocytosine moieties with molecular docking studies. Inorganic Chemistry Communications. 2022;**138**:109263

[23] Taj S, Ahmad M, Ashfaq UA. Exploring of novel 4-hydroxy-2H-benzo [e] [1, 2] thiazine-3-carbohydrazide 1, 1-dioxide derivative as a dual inhibitor of α-glucosidase and α-amylase: Molecular docking, biochemical, enzyme kinetic and in-vivo mouse model study. International Journal of Biological Macromolecules. 2022;**207**:507-521

[24] Rehman SU, Sarwar T, Ishqi HM, Husain MA, Hasan Z, Tabish M. Deciphering the interactions between chlorambucil and calf thymus DNA: A multi-spectroscopic and molecular docking study. Archives of Biochemistry and Biophysics. 2015;**566**:7-14

[25] Emran TB, Rahman MA, Uddin MMN, Dash R, Hossen MF, Mohiuddin M, et al. Molecular docking and inhibition studies on the interactions of Bacopa monnieri's potent phytochemicals against pathogenic Staphylococcus aureus. DARU Journal of Pharmaceutical Sciences. 2015;**23**(1):1-8

[26] Pisano MB, Kumar A, Medda R, Gatto G, Pal R, Fais A, et al. Antibacterial activity and molecular docking studies of a selected series of hydroxy-3-arylcoumarins. Molecules. 2019;**24**(15):2815

[27] Damasceno JPL, Rodrigues RP, Goncalves RDCR, Kitagawa RR. Anti-Helicobacter pylori activity of isocoumarin paepalantine: Morphological and molecular docking analysis. Molecules. 2017;**22**(5):786

[28] Cheng K, Zheng QZ, Qian Y, Shi L, Zhao J, Zhu HL. Synthesis, antibacterial activities and molecular docking studies of peptide and Schiff bases as targeted antibiotics. Bioorganic & Medicinal Chemistry. 2009;**17**(23):7861-7871

[29] Rana KM, Maowa J, Alam A, Dey S, Hosen A, Hasan I, et al. In silico DFT

study, molecular docking, and ADMET predictions of cytidine analogs with antimicrobial and anticancer properties. In Silico Pharmacology. 2021;**9**(1):1-24

[30] Husunet MT, Mısırlı RÇ, Istifli ES, Ila HB. Investigation of the genotoxic effects of patent blue V (E131) in human peripheral lymphocytes and in silico molecular docking. Drug and Chemical Toxicology. 2021:1-7

[31] Liman R, Ali MM, Ciğerci İH, İstifli ES, Sarikurkcu C. Cytotoxic and genotoxic evaluation of copper oxychloride through Allium test and molecular docking studies. Environmental Science and Pollution Research. 2021;**28**(33):44998-45008

[32] Liman R, Ali MM, Istifli ES, Ciğerci İH, Bonciu E. Genotoxic and cytotoxic effects of pethoxamid herbicide on Allium cepa cells and its molecular docking studies to unravel genotoxicity mechanism. Environmental Science and Pollution Research. 2022. DOI: 10.1007/s11356-022-20166-5

[33] Ince Yardimci A, Istifli ES, Acikbas Y, Liman R, Yagmucukardes N, Yilmaz S, et al. Synthesis and characterization of single-walled carbon nanotube: Cyto-genotoxicity in Allium cepa root tips and molecular docking studies. Microscopy Research and Technique. DOI: 10.1002/jemt.24177

[34] Liman R, Kursunlu AN, Ozmen M, Arslan S, Mutlu D, Istifli ES, et al. Synthesis of water soluble symmetric and asymmetric pillar [5] arene derivatives: Cytotoxicity, apoptosis and molecular docking studies. Journal of Molecular Structure. 2022;**1265**:133482

[35] İstifli ES. Preliminary in silico studies of the interactions of certain genotoxic azo dyes with different double-stranded DNA conformations. Colorants. 2022;**1**(2):236-255

[36] Istifli ES, Netz PA, Sihoglu-Tepe A, Husunet MT, Sarikurkcu C, Tepe B. In silico analysis of the interactions of certain flavonoids with the receptor-binding domain of 2019 novel coronavirus and cellular proteases and their pharmacokinetic properties. Journal of Biomolecular Structure & Dynamics. 2022;**40**(6):2460-2474

[37] Istifli ES, Netz PA, Sihoglu-Tepe A, Sarikurkcu C, Tepe B. Understanding the molecular interaction of SARS-CoV-2 spike mutants with ACE2 (angiotensin converting enzyme 2). Journal of Biomolecular Structure & Dynamics. 2021:1-12

[38] Kong R, Yang G, Xue R, Liu M, Wang F, Hu J, et al. COVID-19 Docking Server: A meta server for docking small molecules, peptides and antibodies against potential targets of COVID-19. Bioinformatics. 2020;**36**(20):5109-5111

[39] Sharma AD, Kaur I. Molecular docking studies on Jensenone from eucalyptus essential oil as a potential inhibitor of COVID 19 corona virus infection. arXiv preprint arXiv:2004.00217. 2020

[40] Suravajhala R, Parashar A, Malik B, Nagaraj AV, Padmanaban G, Kavi-Kishor P, et al. Comparative docking studies on curcumin with COVID-19 proteins. Preprints. 2020:2020050439. DOI: 10.20944/preprints202005.0439.v1

[41] Schuller M, Correy GJ, Gahbauer S, Fearon D, Wu T, Díaz RE, et al. Fragment binding to the Nsp3 macrodomain of SARS-CoV-2 identified through crystallographic screening and computational docking. Science Advances. 2021;**7**(16):eabf8711

[42] Wei BQ, Weaver LH, Ferrari AM, Matthews BW, Shoichet BK. Testing a flexible-receptor docking algorithm in a model binding site. Journal of Molecular Biology. 2004;**337**(5):1161-1182

[43] Wong CF. Flexible receptor docking for drug discovery. Expert Opinion on Drug Discovery. 2015;**10**(11):1189-1200

[44] Barril X, Morley SD. Unveiling the full potential of flexible receptor docking using multiple crystallographic structures. Journal of Medicinal Chemistry. 2005;**48**(13):4432-4443

[45] Zhao Y, Sanner MF. FLIPDock: Docking flexible ligands into flexible receptors. Proteins: Structure, Function, and Bioinformatics. 2007;**68**(3):726-737

Section 2

Principles of Molecular Docking

Chapter 2

Fundamentals of Molecular Docking and Comparative Analysis of Protein–Small-Molecule Docking Approaches

Sefika Feyza Maden, Selin Sezer and Saliha Ece Acuner

Abstract

Proteins (e.g., enzymes, receptors, hormones, antibodies, transporter proteins, etc.) seldom act alone in the cell, and their functions rely on their interactions with various partners such as small molecules, other proteins, and/or nucleic acids. Molecular docking is a computational method developed to model these interactions at the molecular level by predicting the 3D structures of complexes. Predicting the binding site and pose of a protein with its partner through docking can help us to unveil protein structure-function relationship and aid drug design in numerous ways. In this chapter, we focus on the fundamentals of protein docking by describing docking methods including search algorithm, scoring, and assessment steps as well as illustrating recent successful applications in drug discovery. We especially address protein–small-molecule (drug) docking by comparatively analyzing available tools implementing different approaches such as ab initio, structure-based, ligand-based (pharmacophore-/shape-based), information-driven, and machine learning approaches.

Keywords: molecular docking, drug design, drug discovery, protein interactions, machine learning

1. Introduction

The molecular machines of the cell, i.e., proteins, are essential to many cellular processes such as signal transduction and cell regulation. Proteins seldom act alone in the cell, but they function through interacting with other small or macromolecules. Therefore, understanding protein interactions at the atomic level is critical to understanding biological processes [1]. Primary structure, i.e., amino acid sequence, of the interacting proteins is a necessary but insufficient source of information at the atomic level. After being synthesized, proteins fold and acquire a stable native structure, i.e., tertiary structure that can be defined in a three-dimensional (3D) plane in order to be functional. It is known that proteins with different sequence information can have similar functional structures, that is, different amino acid sequences can show similar folding trends in 3D space and structure is more conserved than sequence [2]. Therefore, it is crucial to understand the interaction details at the structural level. Proteins physically interact with their partners via non-covalent associations, namely H-bond, hydrophobic, and electrostatic interactions, with the exception of covalent disulfide bridges. These intermolecular physical forces also dominate the protein folding process.

The 3D structure of the macromolecules can be determined using the experimental methods such as X-ray crystallography, nuclear magnetic resonance (NMR), and cryo-EM and then deposited in the Protein Data Bank (PDB) (https://www.rcsb.org). However, there is a huge gap between the number of known protein sequences and structures [3, 4]. Computational modeling approaches that can predict 3D structures of macromolecules can help to bridge this gap. A recent machine learning algorithm developed by DeepMind, called AlphaFold [5], can predict 3D structures of proteins using the sequence information with high accuracy and has been accepted as a breakthrough in the structural biology field. In 1 year, approximately 1 million new structures have been predicted and deposited at AlphaFold Protein Structure Database (https://alphafold.ebi.ac.uk/). In order to have a complete understanding of the proteome, computational techniques are not only needed for modeling single protein structures, but also the interactions between them.

Molecular docking is a method used to predict the structures of proteins in complex with other proteins, nucleic acids, or small molecules. It can be defined as predicting the appropriate low-energy binding pose of the ligand in complex with the target structure, by randomly colliding proteins and their potential partners in space, first creating a rigid complex structure model, and then focusing on the binding sites of that model with flexible interface refinement [6]. Energy minimization of randomly docked conformations in space requires a multidimensional calculation. Initially developed molecular docking method was treating ligands and receptors as rigid bodies without considering any conformational changes [7]. However, interactions between proteins can become quite complex even with small changes in the conformation of the structures [7], and docking algorithms may not physically solve this complex problem correctly [8]. The main factor that creates computational difficulties in docking algorithms is when the protein backbone changes its conformation significantly upon binding [9, 10]. To address this problem, different techniques that consider backbone flexibility have been successfully implemented in docking algorithms [10].

Many diseases today, such as cancer, are likely to be linked to problems in protein-protein interactions and targeting them can therefore enable the development of next-generation therapeutic methods [11]. Modeling the complex structures formed by proteins with other proteins or small molecules holds the key to understand many biological processes such that modeling enzyme-substrate or protein-drug interactions can reveal insights into binding sites/interface regions, function, and mechanism of action. The main protein–small-molecule docking applications in drug discovery include drug repositioning, structure- and ligand-based (pharmacophore–/shape-based) drug design approaches using virtual and reverse screening [11–14]. Today, with the continuously developing technology; targeted drug design, drug target search, evaluation of the side effects of existing drugs, or finding new targets for these drugs can be achieved with the help of molecular modeling and machine learning methods [12]. Deep learning neural network models have strong computational ability on big data and attract attention in structural biology field [15]. There are antibiotic discovery studies using deep neural networks [16] and deep learning studies adapted to drug design [17].

In this chapter, we focus on the protein–small-molecule docking fundamentals and the steps of the docking algorithm and procedure in detail. We then give recent successful applications in drug design and discovery that use different docking approaches, namely virtual screening, reverse screening, and machine learning. Lastly, we comparatively analyze some of the available protein–small-molecule docking tools using the structure of SARS-CoV-2 main protease in complex with a non-covalent inhibitor Jun8-76-3A as a case study.

2. Fundamentals of protein–small-molecule docking

Protein–small-molecule interactions are essential for the sustainability of biological processes such as enzymatic catalysis and overall homeostasis in the body [18]. The engineering of protein–small-molecule interactions is one of the computational approaches used to solve critical problems in biology [18]. Protein–small-molecule docking, i.e., modeling the interaction between chemical compounds and their target protein receptors at the atomic level, is an effective tool in drug design. In the structure-based design of small-molecule drugs, a good estimation of the binding pose is required to clearly demonstrate important interactions and design drugs with increased selectivity and efficacy [19]. The procedures that can be followed and the tools that can be used before, during, and after molecular docking are explained in the following subsections and summarized in **Figure 1**.

2.1 Before docking: molecule preparation

Before starting the docking studies, first of all, the most suitable protein and ligand structures should be selected [20]. There are databases to access the experimentally determined structures of target proteins such as PDB, Uniprot, and Therapeutic Target Database (TTD). If the experimental structure is not available, modeled structures can be obtained from AlphaFold Database or can be modeled

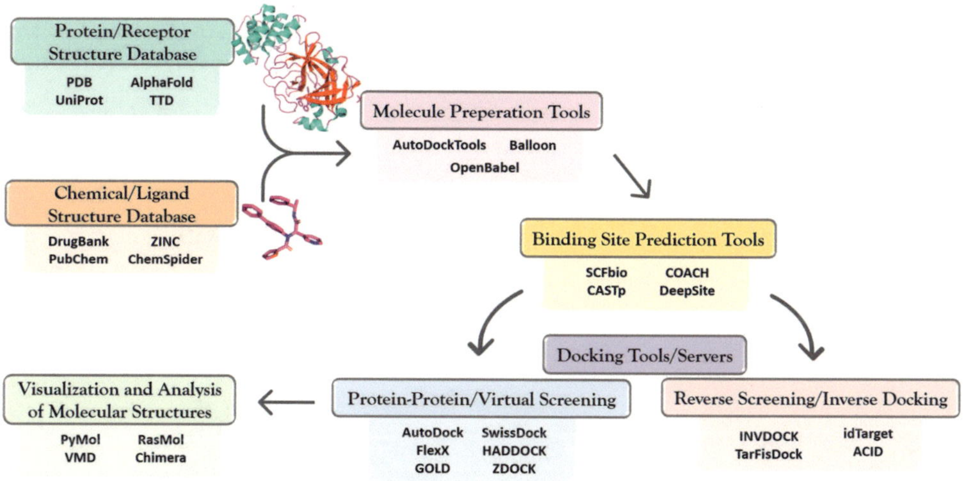

Figure 1.
The procedures that can be followed and the tools that can be used before, during, and after protein-ligand molecular docking in drug design.

using relevant structure modeling software. The most frequently used databases for getting the small-molecule ligand/chemical structures are: DrugBank [21], PubChem [22], ZINC [23], ChEMBL [24], and Chemspider [25] (**Figure 1**). DrugBank, Chemspider, and ZINC databases include more than 500,000, 100 million, and 230 million compounds/drug molecules, respectively.

The molecular docking algorithms may require preliminary preparation of the structures that are obtained in PDB format (lacking H atoms). There are tools available for such preliminary preparations such as Open Babel [26] and AutoDockTools (**Figure 1**) [27].

It is also of crucial importance to guide docking with preliminary information on the binding site. Otherwise, there are no binding site constraints, blind docking takes place, and it is more difficult to detect the correct binding poses when the ligand search space is large. There are various guiding algorithms for active site prediction that can be used when binding sites are not known. Some of them can be listed as: GRID [28], SurfNet [29], COACH [30], SCFbio [31], CASTp [32], DeepSite [33], and PUResNet (**Figure 1**) [34].

The capabilities of docking algorithms can differ from each other, and in this respect, it is important to carefully choose the algorithm to use in accordance with the purpose of the study before starting the docking.

2.2 Docking algorithm steps

There are many approaches and algorithms for molecular docking, based on different parameters, and they aim to perform the protein-ligand docking with the best performance [12]. The steps of molecular docking algorithms can be summarized as follows: molecule flexibility, conformational search algorithms (ligand sampling), and scoring functions (**Figure 2**) [12, 35].

2.2.1 Molecule flexibility

During molecular docking, structures can be considered rigid or flexible. Rigid docking takes into account only the translation and rotation degrees of freedom. Providing flexibility means also considering the rotation about single bonds so that they have the same bond lengths and angles but different torsion angles. Although

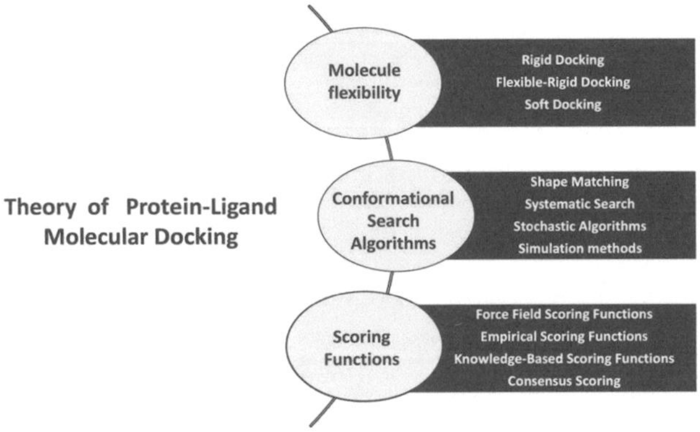

Figure 2.
Methods for protein-ligand molecular docking.

flexible docking approach is more realistic than rigid docking, when there are many rotatable bonds, the ligand conformational search space becomes so large that it is difficult to find the correct binding pose with the lowest binding free energy (global minimum solution). Some algorithms, such as HADDOCK [36], first treat the structures as rigid to increase time efficiency and then perform flexibility improvements on the poses of molecules with the best energy scores. Molecular docking software can be grouped according to the flexibility treatments of molecules such as Rigid Docking, Semi-Flexible Docking, and Soft Docking [35, 37].

In rigid docking, protein and ligand molecules are treated as rigid entities [37, 38]. During docking, the positions of the molecules change without losing their shape [37], i.e., only translation and rotation but no conformational degrees of freedom are considered.

Semi-flexible docking is based on the principle of keeping the protein structure rigid and letting the ligand structure be flexible by allowing rotatable bonds. Thus, various conformational poses of the ligand on the protein are sampled [35, 37, 38]. It gives more accurate results than rigid docking [37].

In soft docking, van der Waals interactions between atoms are softened, making the structures of both receptor and ligand molecules implicitly flexible as overlap is allowed to a small extent [39, 40]. Soft docking process is carried out realistically by ensuring that both the protein and the ligand are rotatable as in their natural states [37, 38]. It is an advantageous method due to its computational efficiency and ease of application [35, 37].

2.2.2 Conformational search algorithms

Conformational search algorithms can identify different conformational orientations (poses) of the ligand sampled around the experimentally determined active site or other binding sites on the protein [35, 41, 42]. These algorithms are generally classified as: shape matching, systematic, stochastic, and simulation methods [35, 38, 43].

Shape matching algorithms have the advantage of speed over other algorithms [35, 44] and adopt a sampling principle in which the conformation of the ligand should be structurally complementary to the protein binding site [38]. It ensures that the ligand is positioned in such a way that best complements the molecular surface of the binding site on the protein [35]. Some example software using shape matching are: DOCK [45], FLOG [46], EUDOC [47], Surflex [48], LibDOCK [49], SANDOCK [50], and MDock [51].

Using systematic search algorithms, a large number of possible binding poses can be obtained by gradually changing the degrees of freedom of the ligands [35, 52] toward the direction of minimum energy. Systematic search algorithms can be divided into two as exhaustive search and fragmentation (incremental structure) [35, 41, 53]. Exhaustive search algorithm is based on systematically generating flexible ligand conformations by rotating the rotatable bonds in the ligand [35]. If the number of rotatable bonds is large, there is a combinatorial explosion in the number of poses, i.e., the search space, so that some filtering and optimization procedures are applied for practical purposes [35]. Glide [54] and FRED [55] are example docking software using exhaustive conformational search algorithms. In the fragmentation method, the ligand is divided into smaller fragments, each fragment is placed and augmented at the binding site gradually through covalent bonding to the previous one [35]. DOCK [56], LUDI [57], FlexX [58], and eHiTs [59] are example software using fragmentation.

The algorithms used in stochastic search methods are more efficient but do not guarantee an accurate result as they are based on generating random ligand conformations, and therefore, the docking process is iterative in these algorithms [41, 44]. Monte Carlo, swarm optimization, evolutionary algorithms, and Tabu search methods are among the most used stochastic algorithms [35, 38, 52]. Example software using stochastic conformational search method include AutoDock [60], GOLD [61], DockThor [62], and MolDock [63].

Simulations of the obtained ligand poses (simulation methods) represent protein and ligand flexibility better than the other algorithms but have a slow flow and can make insufficient sampling [38, 44]. For this reason, they are used as a complement to other conformational search methods [38].

2.2.3 Scoring functions

In the previously described conformational search step, many structures are created and most of them should be eliminated by selecting the biologically appropriate structures. Therefore, the possible poses created by conformational search algorithms are evaluated and ranked by using a scoring function [35]. The scoring function is a measure to evaluate the docking poses obtained [35, 38, 52] in terms of their binding free energies [11, 44, 64].

With the scoring functions that estimate the binding energies of the created complex structures, various physicochemical properties should be evaluated in order to distinguish good results from the bad ones. These physicochemical properties can be intermolecular interactions, desolvation from solvent, electrostatic and entropic effects, etc. [65]. As the number of evaluated parameters increases, the accuracy of the scoring function will increase; but the computational load will also increase. Therefore, scoring functions with ideal efficiency, especially when working with large ligand sets, are those that are balanced in terms of accuracy and speed [11]. The scoring functions can be classified as: force-field-based, empirical, knowledge-based, and consensus scoring.

The Force Field Scoring Function (FFSF) is designed to work with multiple force fields such as AMBER [66], CHARMM [67], GROMOS [68], and OPLS [69] individually or in combination. The designed FFSFs estimate the free energy of ligand binding by considering van der Waals energy terms such as electrostatic interactions and hydrogen bonds [35, 38].

Empirical scoring functions use simpler energy terms to estimate the free energy of ligand binding such as hydrogen bonds and ionic interaction, and they can be calculated more easily and faster than FFSFs [35, 38, 52]. Some examples of empirical scoring functions are GlideScore [54], PLP [70], LigScore [71], LUDI [72], SCORE [73], and X-Score [74].

Knowledge-based scoring functions use statistical analysis of protein-ligand complex structures to derive protein-ligand distance [44]. These functions can show high performance in a short time [52]. They can also model some uncommon interactions, such as sulfur-aromatic, that other functions do not address [44].

Consensus scoring function, not a specific scoring system, aims at an effective scoring with a combination of multiple scoring functions with the idea of minimizing the possible error margins of existing scoring systems [35, 38, 44].

2.3 After docking: evaluation of the results

After performing protein-ligand docking studies, the accuracy of pose estimations needs to be evaluated [41, 52]. The best way to evaluate the docking algorithm is to compare the predicted binding pose of the ligand with position of the reference ligand in the experimentally determined structure, if possible. The structural comparison is quantified by using root mean squared deviation (RMSD) (Eq. 1), with the unit of Å [41, 75]. It is preferred that this value is between 2 and 4 Å or less for a good docking. RMSD calculations are simple, but this metric is not normalized to number of atoms and therefore should not be considered as an absolute measure [76]. As a more systematic approach, in order to ensure the consistency of the docking algorithm used, it should be checked whether the same poses are obtained by repeating the docking process [52] at least 50 times and clustering the poses of the side chains and references according to a certain threshold value [77]. With this method, whether the docking algorithm correctly and consistently creates a pose in the right position can be determined [41, 44, 78].

$$RMSD = \sqrt{\frac{1}{N} + \sum_{i=1}^{N} \left(x_{ai} - x_{bi}\right)^2 + \left(y_{ai} - y_{bi}\right)^2 + \left(z_{ai} - z_{bi}\right)^2} \quad (1)$$

Eq. (1) Root mean squared deviation for the coordinates of two molecules, a and b, with N atoms.

Modeling successes and capabilities of docking algorithms are being evaluated in a competition called CAPRI (Critical Assessment of Protein Interactions) (https://www.capri-docking.org/) since 2001 [79, 80]. Experimentally determined complex structures that have not yet been published in PDB are submitted to CAPRI and without knowing the experimental structure of the complex, the participants try to predict the most similar structure to the experimentally determined complex structure through docking algorithms [79]. A solution set of 10 models is presented to the CAPRI committee for evaluation based on the geometry similarity and biological relevance of the predicted complex structures. The results of CAPRI show very good predictions for easy targets with simple conformational changes, but rather worse ones for difficult targets with conformational changes upon binding [9].

3. Molecular docking approaches and applications in drug design

Computational methods have become an important part of the drug discovery process with increasing accuracy of algorithms. Various docking methods based on different algorithms are constantly being developed to determine the structural relationships of potential drug molecules and their targets [44]. In addition, studies in this area shed light on the candidate drugs in terms of the pharmacodynamic properties, affinity, and selectivity [11]. The main molecular docking applications in drug discovery include drug repositioning (repurposing), structure- and ligand-based drug design approaches using virtual and reverse screening [11–14].

Drug repositioning seeks out new targets for natural compounds, drugs currently in use, or candidate ligands to reveal their unknown therapeutic potentials [81]. Many successful repositioning studies are available in the literature [81–83]. Virtual screening (VS) and reverse screening (RS) techniques are frequently used in drug discovery and repositioning. VS offers a more effective and rational approach compared with traditional methods [36]. The atomic-level analyzable results presented to us by virtual screening studies guide us in understanding the function of the target and in new drug discoveries [5, 36, 55]. In the RS approach, interest is on a single ligand molecule, and there is a search for a biological target for this molecule [12]. Unlike virtual screening (VS), the search library consists of potential target receptors. RS approach has the potential to lead studies such as testing toxicity or side effects of the existing drugs [38]. The potential side effects of a drug need to be evaluated in the drug discovery process. Molecular docking studies can offer an important perspective in this regard, and there are inverse (reverse) docking studies that provide bioactivity data by detecting off-target bindings [25]. Lastly, the subclasses of Artificial Intelligence (AI): Machine Learning (ML) and Deep Learning (DL) methods have significant contributions in pharmaceutical industry [84]. AI can be applied to different steps such as drug design with VS, *de novo* generation of drug molecules, and computational planning of drug synthesis [85]. Recent developments are promising that molecular docking methods may benefit from the machine learning methods more in the future [84].

3.1 Virtual screening

Virtual screening (VS) approach uses a target receptor and a library of small molecules. Libraries can be created manually, or already existing libraries can be used. The library consists of a large number of chemically diverse bioactive small molecules with a high probability of binding to the receptor. This virtual computing technique is considered as the *in silico* equivalent of *in vitro* methods such as high-throughput screening (HTS) [11]. VS is preferred as a guide in scientific studies because its success rate is 400 times higher [86], less costly, faster, and requires less labor compared with high-throughput screening methods [87]. VS studies aim to reduce a large number of potential drug candidates to manageable numbers applying various filters. The biggest challenge in VS is the detection of false negatives [19].

Ligand-based VS methods conduct research by identifying common properties of compound sequences, such as molecular volume and protonation state [11]. In addition to chemical similarity [88] and rule-based [89] software included in filtration strategies, there are also various software such as freely add-on pharmacophore and quantitative structure-activity relationship (QSAR) models [87, 90]. The most commonly used ligand-based virtual screening method is the QSAR method. Ligand-based VS does not contain structural information about the receptor, it only scans using receptor sites known to be active and tries to detect active ligand molecules [85].

Structure-based VS methods are often used when the receptor has different conformations. The aim is to predict receptor binding affinity by processing structural information using a variety of techniques, such as binding site similarity and pharmacophore mapping. By estimating the different binding modes, the molecules are sorted for evaluation [11]. Analysis of the predicted poses can be done manually using visualization programs. It has been reported that nAPOLI, a web server developed in recent years, analyzes results automatically [91].

Structure-based pharmacophore generation is one of the most frequently used methods for small molecules in the virtual screening method. Here, 3D pharmacophore model interfaces of the scaffolds of the ligands are created, and ligands that will adapt to the binding site and provide the desired bioactivity are selected. Some of the programs that use pharmacophore modeling are HipHop [92], PHASE [93], MOE, which are commercial, SCAMPI [94], PharmaGist [95], ALADDIN [96], which are suitable for academic use.

A recent example of VS application on the non-structural protein of SARS-CoV-2, nsp1, one of the virulence factors causing viral infection, is by G. O. Timo *et al.* [74]. They estimated the exact pattern of nsp1 interaction through molecular simulation studies and analyzed 8694 potential inhibitors from the DrugBank database using the virtual screening method and proposed 16 inhibitor molecules with the best binding energy scores [74]. There is another recent study on the transcription factor BRF2, which is among the therapeutic targets as its upregulation is observed in the formation of various types of cancer, but there is no available specific drug targeting BRF2. By performing drug repositioning through virtual screening of drug molecules that are potential candidates for BRF2 inhibition, Rashidieh *et al.* found that the bexarotene molecule led to a serious decrease in the proliferation of this type of cancer cells [97].

3.2 Reverse screening

Reverse screening (RS) is also called inverse docking, reverse docking, inverse virtual screening, or target screening. Libraries are more limited for target hunting and profiling [12] and can be created manually using the most common accessible databases such as PDB [98] and TTD [12, 99]. But this process requires a long preparation time and effort. There are various algorithms used to detect interactions by reverse screening. Some web platforms (INVDOCK [100], idTarget [101], ACTP [102], etc.) have been developed for reverse docking, which use libraries prepared for specific diseases and docked using programs such as standard AutoDock and AutoDock Vina [12].

A recently developed Consensus Reverse Docking System (CRDS) detects potential binding sites by screening approximately 5200 candidate proteins for the ligand molecule using three different scoring methods [103]. In another example, Stepanova *et al.* tested the antimicrobial activity against *Mycobacterium tuberculosis* strain by reverse screening for chemicals that had been successful in experimental studies and determined the most appropriate target as aspartate 1-decarboxylase by performing docking studies using 35 different target protein structures [104]. Reverse screening was also used for Bazedoxifene, an FDA-approved drug for the prevention of postmenopausal osteoporosis, and Xiao *et al.* defined the inhibitory power of Bazedoxifene on IL-6/GP130 signaling pathway (critical for cancer survival) by using computational techniques and confirmed the result with *in vivo* studies [83].

3.3 Machine-learning-based approaches

Machine learning techniques take information from biological data and make predictions about them, thus contributing to building a structural model [9]. Once a model is built, it must be improved so that the state with the lowest potential energy (global minimum) can be reached. Global minimum means a stable and sterically acceptable structure, and reaching it without being stuck at the local minima is very important in the field of bioinformatics and computational structural biology. A recent machine learning algorithm developed by DeepMind, called AlphaFold [5], implements deep learning and can predict 3D structures of proteins using the sequence information with high accuracy and has been accepted as a breakthrough in the structural biology field.

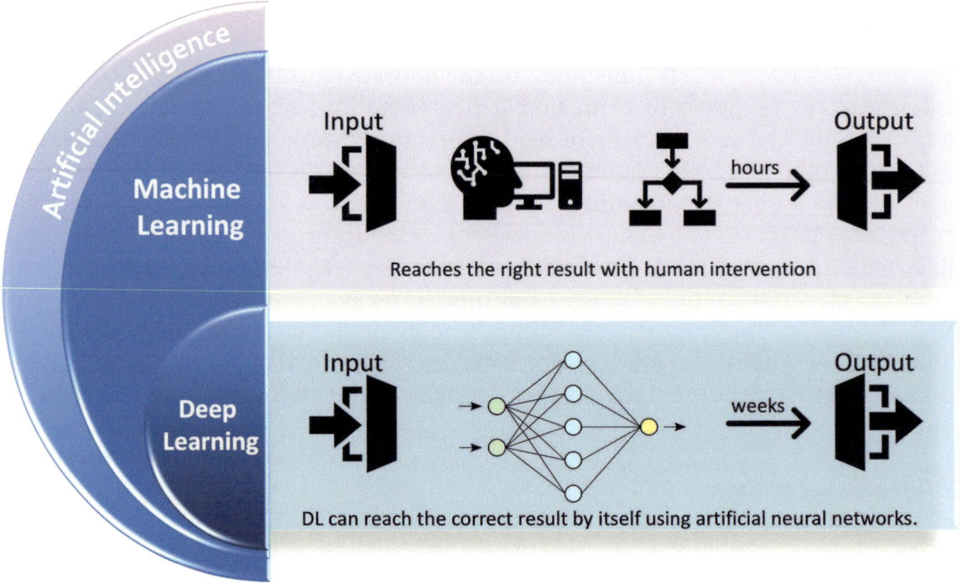

Figure 3.
Schematic illustration of artificial intelligence subfields: Machine learning and deep learning.

Machine learning makes classifications by learning on datasets and needs human intervention to evaluate possible outcomes. Deep learning is a more advanced model having the neural network with ability to decide the right result without human intervention (**Figure 3**). Machine learning can use supervised or unsupervised learning. Supervised learning performs machine learning on datasets that we know about, whereas unsupervised learning detects and labels similarities and orientations in a created cluster [38, 90].

The training set used in machine learning constitutes the performance of the algorithm. Machine learning studies in the field of virtual screening are generally focused on improving the performance of the scoring function [85]. Studies have shown that working with small subsets of the same family, which consists of similar structures, gives better scoring results rather than working with large data from different complexes [105]. Working with subsets of interest is also a better approach in terms of computational requirements [38].

Machine learning and deep learning can describe more diverse data than other computational systems and can be representative of structural biology. Nonparametric machine learning has great potential to be the next step in computer-based programming to improve the accuracy of molecular docking studies [41]. Machine learning can be used to refine predetermined function data as well as provide high-quality data to complement pharmaceutical discovery research and development.

4. Case study: comparison of docking tools

As a case study for comparing different protein-ligand docking tools, the crystal structure of the SARS-CoV-2 (COVID-19) main protease in complex with its non-covalent inhibitor Jun8-76-3A (PDB ID: 7KX5) is used as the experimental reference structure to evaluate the accuracies of the complex structures predicted using

AutoDock Vina, HADDOCK, and SwissDock programs and changing some of the parameters to test their effects on prediction capabilities. The inhibitor in the experimental protein structure is removed and then molecular docking is performed using the initial coordinates of the main protease structure of SARS-CoV-2 and its inhibitor Jun8-76-3A, separately.

4.1 Docking with AutoDock Vina

AutoDock is a free software that predicts the binding compatibility of small ligands to macromolecule targets with a flexible-rigid (semi-flexible) docking approach [27]. It uses a grid-based method to place the ligand in the active region determined on the macromolecule [106]. AutoDockTools (http://mgltools.scripps.edu/downloads) is the user interface to produce and examine grid information required for the preparation of the protein and ligand structures in the relevant format and the configuration file [27].

As a docking input in AutoDock Vina, a configuration file, which contains the coordinate information of the protein and ligand structures and the ligand-binding region on the receptor, is required. For docking the case study ligand to the receptor using AutoDock Vina, the structure file was downloaded from RCSB PDB database (https://www.rcsb.org) in .pdb format (PDB ID:7KX5). AutoDockTools (v1.5.6) interface was used to prepare input files, such that, water molecules in the relevant protein structure were deleted, polar H bonds were added to the structure and both the receptor and ligand structures were saved in .pdbqt file format. After preparing the ligand and protein structures, the most important input information for AutoDock is the docking parameter. The docking parameter involves determining the coordinates of the ligand-binding region on the target protein. While determining the docking parameter, if the binding region on the protein is not known, blind docking can be performed by putting the whole protein in the grid box (**Figure 4A**), or a small grid box can be placed in the specific known/predicted ligand-binding region on the protein (**Figure 4B**). Lastly, after determining the region on the protein where the ligand is to be bound by using the "grid box" in AutoDockTools, the protein coordinates were

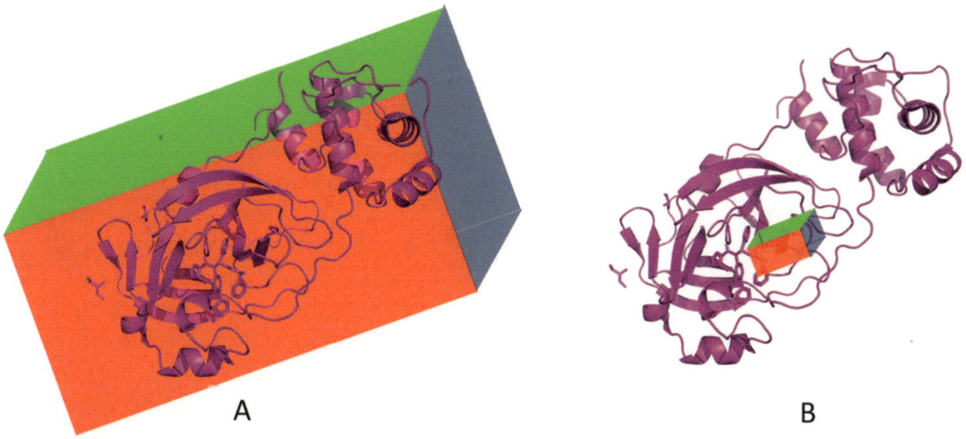

Figure 4.
Grid box usage in docking: (A) blind docking with a grid box of size: $44 \times 72 \times 68$ *and center coordinates: 10.711, 0.0, 3.782, (B) specific docking with a grid box of size:* $14 \times 14 \times 16$ *and center coordinates: 10.735, −2.409, 21.173.*

Mode	Specific docking Affinity (kcal/mol)				Blind docking Affinity (kcal/mol)			
	Rep1	Rep 2	Rep 3	AVG	Rep1	Rep2	Rep3	AVG
1	−8.9	−8.8	−8.9	−8.9	−8.9	−8.9	−9.0	−8.9
2	−7.3	−8.7	−7.3	−7.8	−8.2	−8.2	−8.3	−8.2
3	−7.2	−7.2	−7.3	−7.2	−8.1	−8.0	−8.1	−8.1
4	−6.8	−7.0	−7.0	−6.9	−7.9	−7.8	−8.0	−7.9
5	−6.8	−6.9	−7.0	−6.9	−7.9	−7.5	−8.0	−7.8
6	−6.8	−6.8	−6.9	−6.8	−7.7	−7.4	−7.8	−7.6
7	−6.7	−6.5	−6.8	−6.7	−7.7	−7.4	−7.8	−7.6
8	−6.4	−6.4	−6.8	−6.5	−7.6	−7.2	−7.6	−7.5
9	−6.3	−6.4	−6.7	−6.4	−7.5	−6.9	−7.4	−7.3

Table 1.
Specific and blind docking studies with AutoDock were repeated three times.

specified in the input configuration file. Preparing all the required inputs, docking was performed using AutoDock Vina by repeating each docking process three times in order to observe the consistency of the algorithm (**Table 1**).

In order to examine the accuracy of the docking results, the poses obtained from AutoDock Vina were aligned with the original PDB structure by using the PyMol program [107]. When the energies of the poses predicted with specific docking (i.e., using specific grid on the binding site) and blind docking are compared, although the energy scores of the blind docking results are better, the comparison of the poses with the reference ligand shows that the most accurate binding is achieved with specific docking (**Figure 5**). Alignment of the first poses (with the lowest energy score) predicted with specific docking (green) and blind docking studies (blue) with the reference ligand (red) shows that the specific docking pose was in a more similar position with the reference ligand (green vs. red), than the blind docking pose (blue vs. red).

4.2 Docking with HADDOCK

An integrative platform called High Ambiguity-Driven biomolecular DOCKing (HADDOCK) is used for molecular docking of two or more molecules [108] and is a popular algorithm [36]. Although it is mainly suitable for protein-protein interactions, it can also be applied to model the protein–small-molecule complexes [109]. HADDOCK automatically decides the most suitable configuration of the ligand according to the given restrictions [108]. Protein-protein docking is more complex than protein–small-molecule docking, as the proteins are flexible and the conformational space is larger [110].

HADDOCK does not require CPU and allows the user to see all the docking steps from start to finish. It should be noted that the success of HADDOCK studies is directly related with the amount of data entered into the system [36]. HADDOCK allows processing different types of molecules with the help of different platforms such as WHATIF, ProDRG, PDB. There is no need to create different conformer

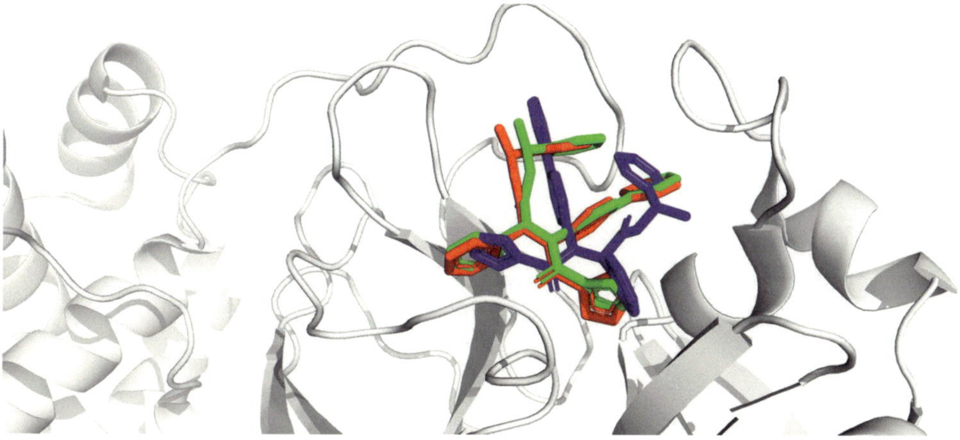

Figure 5.
Crystal SARS-CoV-2 main protease structure (white, PDB ID: 7KX5_chain (A) in complex with the blind docking (blue), specific docking (green) poses predicted with AutoDock Vina and the reference ligand Jun8-76-3A inhibitor (red, PDB ID: 7KX5_chain B). This figure was drawn with PyMol 2.5.2.

sequences as the system selects the most compatible conformers based on the shape constraints. With restriction files, we can set clear target sites, binding distances, or select active or passive residues (areas that are likely to interact). Defining semi-flexible regions is also allowed.

HADDOCK algorithm consists of three stages: rigid-body minimization and randomization of orientations (it0), semi-flexible simulated annealing in torsion angle space (it1), and refinement in 3D space with explicit solvent (water) (https://www.bonvinlab.org/education/HADDOCK-protein-protein-basic/). it0 stage treats structures as rigid solids and 1000 poses with the best score are selected. it1 optimizes orientations by allowing different docking poses from it0 to have different flexible regions defined. Two-hundred models with the best energy pass to the final stage. In the final step, a complex solvent medium (DMSO or water) is considered to improve the interaction energy and the final models are automatically aggregated.

To dock the case study inhibitor-protein complex (PDB ID:7XK5), the guideline tutorial (HADDOCK small-molecule binding site screening protocol) [111] was followed and two different approaches were tested: (i) using an unambiguous (distance) restraint file, indicating the target that should bind the ligand, (ii) by defining the active and passive residues. This case study consists of a pre-docking for the detection of the binding region and a second docking for the detection of binding pose.

First, we tested HADDOCK's accuracy of binding site detection. Two different binding sites were detected in the top 10 clusters with the best energy scores and 70% (7 out of 10) of the clusters were in the correct binding site (**Figure 6A**). Secondly, an ambiguous and unambiguous restraint file was created by identifying the region with the highest number of interactions between the ligand and the receptor. The restraint files can be created manually or using the link in the protocol. However, it may be necessary to make corrections in the distance restraints. The structure with the best energy is visualized in **Figure 6B**. Secondly, active and passive residues were defined on the system, and the pose with the best energy result is visualized in **Figure 6C**. HADDOCK results are summarized in **Table 2**.

Comparison of the results shows that HADDOCK is successful in detecting the binding site. However, according to the results obtained in the second stage, the

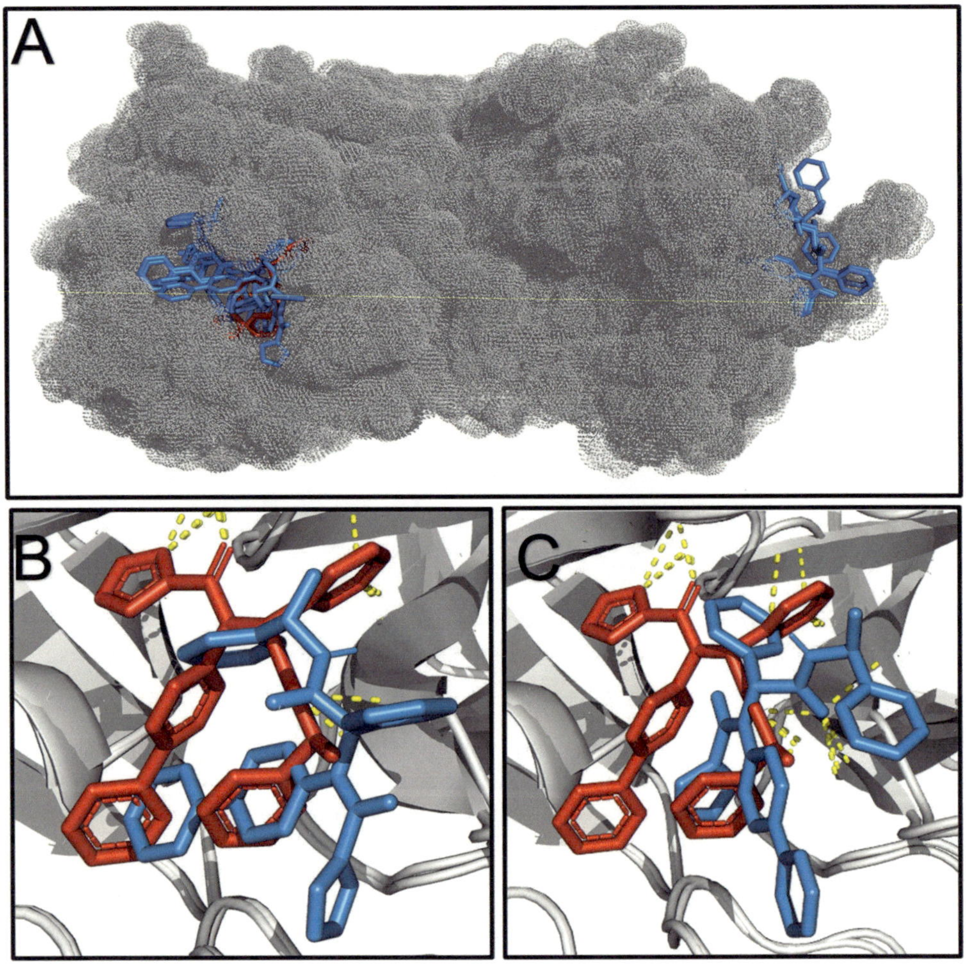

Figure 6.
Crystal SARS-CoV-2 main protease structure (gray, PDB ID: 7KX5_chain (A) in complex with the docking poses (blue) predicted with HADDOCK and reference ligand Jun8-76-3A inhibitor (red, PDB ID: 7KX5_chain B). A. Top 10 clusters for binding site determination. B. Pose with the best energy using ambiguous/unambiguous restraints. C. Pose With the best energy using active/passive restraints. This figure was drawn with PyMol 2.5.2.

algorithm was not successful enough to find the correct conformation of the ligand in binding site. Defining ambiguous/unambiguous restraint files or selecting active and passive residues did not make a significant contribution in detecting the correct binding pose (**Figure 6B** and **C**). Docking with both approaches was repeated several times and no significant similarity was detected.

4.3 Docking with SwissDock

SwissDock is a database to improve protein–small-molecule docking using amino acid sequence information from genome projects. Moreover, it is a web browser and programmatic interface that enables creating three-dimensional protein models from protein amino acid sequences [112]. It also has user interfaces such as Swiss-Pdb Viewer (DeepView) to simultaneously analyze several proteins [113]. Using the SwissDock web server, the starting crystal structures of the target proteins can

	Binding site detection	Ambiguous/ Unambiguous restraints	Active/passive restraints
HADDOCK score	−53.4 ± 1.5	−52.1 ± 0.5	−21.9 ± 2.7
Cluster size	69	5	13
RMSD from the overall lowest-energy structure	0.3 ± 0.2	0.1 ± 0.1	0.2 ± 0.0
Van der Waals energy	−40.3 ± 1.2	−41.6 ± 0.2	−32.4 ± 4.5
Electrostatic energy	−22.1 ± 1.9	−15.2 ± 6.0	−25.8 ± 7.3
Desolvation energy	−10.9 ± 2.5	−9.0 ± 0.2	−6.7 ± 0.3
Restraints violation energy	0.0 ± 0.00	0.7 ± 0.2	198.5 ± 78.0
Buried Surface Area	795.4 ± 21.9	781.6 ± 5.2	783.0 ± 9.4
Z-Score	−1.7	−2.4	−1.3

Table 2.
HADDOCK results.

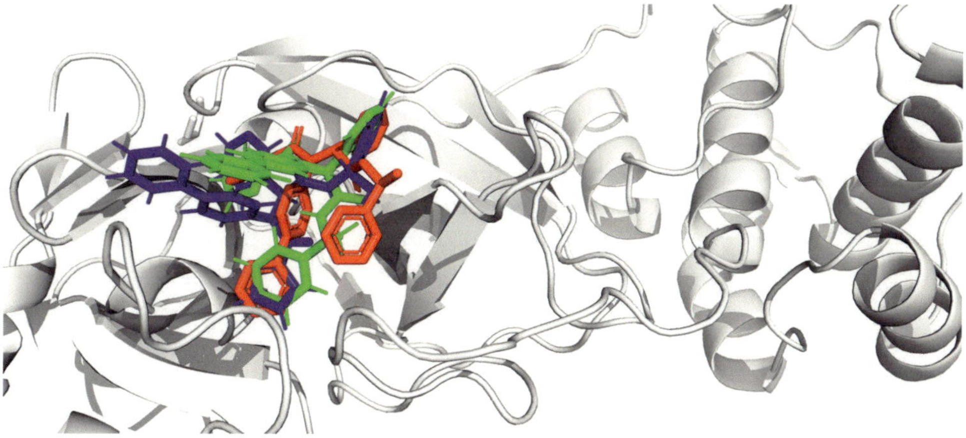

Figure 7.
Crystal SARS-CoV-2 main protease structure (white, PDB ID: 7KX5_chain (A) in complex with the blind docking (blue), specific docking (green) poses predicted by SwissDock and the reference ligand Jun8-76-3A inhibitor (red, PDB ID: 7KX5_chain B). This figure was drawn with PyMol 2.5.2.

be searched and fetched from protein and ligand structure databases. If there is no crystal structure available to compare, it provides homology modeling of the studied protein. During the docking process, the user does not have to do any calculations because all calculations are handled by the server side [112]. As a docking constraint, the ligand binding region can be defined or blind docking can be applied with no information.

Using the case study, both specific and blind dockings were performed on the SwissDock server, and the results were compared. The server presented 256 poses. The best scores obtained by specific docking (green) blind docking (blue) were −9.88 and −9.35 kcal/mol, respectively (**Figure 7**). Although both of the predicted poses did not show the same conformation with the reference ligand, it was observed that the pose obtained from the specific docking (green) was more similar to the reference ligand (red) (**Figure 7**).

5. Conclusions

Molecular docking is a computational method that predicts the 3D structures of receptor-ligand complexes. Modeling the atomic details of the ligand pose with the receptor protein by molecular docking can assist in understanding protein structure-function relationship and in drug design studies in several ways. Computational modeling approaches complement and/or lead experiments by eliminating irrelevant drug candidates and selecting the ones with the best binding properties. With the continuously developing technology, there are many different approaches and algorithms for molecular docking studies, and they are successfully used in therapeutic applications such as targeted drug design, drug target search, evaluation of the side effects of existing drugs, or finding new targets for these drugs.

The crystal structure of the SARS-CoV-2 (COVID-19) main protease in complex with its non-covalent inhibitor Jun8-76-3A (PDB ID: 7KX5) was used as an experimental reference case study to compare and evaluate the prediction accuracies of AutoDock Vina, HADDOCK, and SwissDock programs as well as to test the effects of some parameters on their prediction capabilities. One of the main observations is that the ligand poses with the lowest binding energy scores are not necessarily the best solution. Therefore, docking results should always be evaluated in terms of biological relevance. Moreover, when *a priori* information about the ligand-binding site is included as grid box placement and size in AutoDock Vina and as ligand binding residues in SwissDock, the binding accuracy is improved significantly.

In summary, before starting the molecular docking, it is of crucial importance to obtain detailed information on the target protein and ligand from various sources and servers and to decide which docking algorithm to use. Moreover, the top predicted poses with the best scores should not be unquestioningly accepted as the best solutions but further structural analyses and evaluations should be incorporated in the decision process.

Acknowledgements

We would like to thank dear Merve DEMİR AKYÜZ and Merve YÜCETÜRK (a.k.a Merves), who are fourth-year undergraduate students at Molecular Biology and Genetics Department of Istanbul Medeniyet University, for their contribution to the writing of the introduction section.

Author details

Sefika Feyza Maden, Selin Sezer and Saliha Ece Acuner*
Department of Bioengineering and Science and Advanced Technologies Research Center (BILTAM), Istanbul Medeniyet University, Istanbul, Turkey

*Address all correspondence to: ece.ozbababacan@medeniyet.edu.tr

References

[1] Russell RB, Alber F, Aloy P, Davis FP, Korkin D, Pichaud M, et al. A structural perspective on protein–protein interactions. Current Opinion in Structural Biology. 2004;**14**(3):313-324

[2] Sadowski MI, Jones DT. The sequence–structure relationship and protein function prediction. Current Opinion in Structural Biology. 2009;**19**(3):357-362

[3] Petrey D, Honig B. Structural bioinformatics of the interactome. Annual Review in Biophysics. 2014;**43**(1):193-210

[4] Stein A, Mosca R, Aloy P. Three-dimensional modeling of protein interactions and complexes is going 'omics. Current Opinion in Structural Biology. 2011;**21**(2):200-208

[5] Senior AW, Evans R, Jumper J, Kirkpatrick J, Sifre L, Green T, et al. Improved protein structure prediction using potentials from deep learning. Nature. 2020;**577**(7792):706-710

[6] Andrusier N, Mashiach E, Nussinov R, Wolfson HJ. Principles of flexible protein-protein docking. Proteins. 2008;**73**(2):271-289

[7] Bonvin AM. Flexible protein–protein docking. Current Opinion in Structural Biology. 2006;**16**(2):194-200

[8] Vakser IA. Protein-protein docking: From Interaction to Interactome. Biophysical Journal. 2014;**107**(8):1785-1793

[9] Harmalkar A, Gray JJ. Advances to tackle backbone flexibility in protein docking. Current Opinion in Structural Biology. 2021;**67**:178-186

[10] Wang C, Bradley P, Baker D. Protein–protein docking with backbone flexibility. Journal of Molecular Biology. 2007;**373**(2):503-519

[11] Ferreira L, dos Santos R, Oliva G, Andricopulo A. Molecular docking and structure-based drug design strategies. Molecules. 2015;**20**(7):13384-13421

[12] Pinzi L, Rastelli G. Molecular docking: Shifting paradigms in drug discovery. IJMS. 2019;**20**(18):4331

[13] March-Vila E, Pinzi L, Sturm N, Tinivella A, Engkvist O, Chen H, et al. On the integration of in silico drug design methods for drug repurposing. Frontiers in Pharmacology. 2017;**23**(8):298

[14] Wilson GL, Lill MA. Integrating structure-based and ligand-based approaches for computational drug design. Future Medicinal Chemistry. 2011;**3**(6):735-750

[15] Anighoro A. Deep learning in structure-based drug design. Methods in Molecular Biology. 2022;**2390**:261-271

[16] Stokes JM, Yang K, Swanson K, Jin W, Cubillos-Ruiz A, Donghia NM, et al. A deep learning approach to antibiotic discovery. Cell. 2020;**180**(4):688-702.e13

[17] Elton DC, Boukouvalas Z, Fuge MD, Chung PW. Deep learning for molecular design—a review of the state of the art. Molecular System and Design Engineering. 2019;**4**(4):828-849

[18] Allison B, Combs S, DeLuca S, Lemmon G, Mizoue L, Meiler J. Computational design of protein-small molecule interfaces. Journal of Structural Biology. 2014;**185**(2):193-202

[19] Śledź P, Caflisch A. Protein structure-based drug design: From docking to molecular dynamics. Current Opinion in Structural Biology. 2018;**48**:93-102

[20] Guterres H, Im W. Improving protein-ligand docking results with high-throughput molecular dynamics simulations. Journal of Chemical Model. 2020;**60**(4):2189-2198

[21] Wishart DS. DrugBank: A comprehensive resource for in silico drug discovery and exploration. Nucleic Acids Research. 2006;**34**(90001):D668-D672

[22] Li Q, Cheng T, Wang Y, Bryant SH. PubChem as a public resource for drug discovery. Drug Discovery Today. 2010;**15**(23-24):1052-1057

[23] Irwin JJ, Sterling T, Mysinger MM, Bolstad ES, Coleman RG. ZINC: A Free Tool to Discover Chemistry for Biology. Journal of Chemical Information and Modeling. 2012;**52**(7):1757-1768

[24] Gaulton A, Bellis LJ, Bento AP, Chambers J, Davies M, Hersey A, et al. ChEMBL: A large-scale bioactivity database for drug discovery. Nucleic Acids Research. 2012;**40**(D1):D1100-D1107

[25] Pence HE, Williams A. ChemSpider: An online chemical information resource. Journal of Chemical Education. 2010;**87**(11):1123-1124

[26] O'Boyle NM, Banck M, James CA, Morley C, Vandermeersch T, Hutchison GR. Open Babel: An open chemical toolbox. Journal of Cheminformatics. 2011;**3**(1):33

[27] Morris GM, Huey R, Lindstrom W, Sanner MF, Belew RK, Goodsell DS, et al. AutoDock4 and AutoDockTools4: Automated docking with selective receptor flexibility. Journal of Computational Chemistry. 2009;**30**(16):2785-2791

[28] Goodford PJ. A computational procedure for determining energetically favorable binding sites on biologically important macromolecules. Journal of Medicinal Chemistry. 1985;**28**(7):849-857

[29] Laskowski RA. SURFNET: A program for visualizing molecular surfaces, cavities, and intermolecular interactions. Journal of Molecular Graphics. 1995;**13**(5):323-330

[30] Yang J, Roy A, Zhang Y. Protein-ligand binding site recognition using complementary binding-specific substructure comparison and sequence profile alignment. Bioinformatics. 2013;**29**(20):2588-2595

[31] Narang P, Bhushan K, Bose S, Jayaram B. Protein structure evaluation using an all-atom energy based empirical scoring function. Journal of Biomolecular Structure & Dynamics. 2006;**23**(4):385-406

[32] Binkowski TA, Naghibzadeh S, Liang J. CASTp: Computed Atlas of Surface Topography of proteins. Nucleic Acids Research. 2003;**31**(13):3352-3355

[33] Jiménez J, Doerr S, Martínez-Rosell G, Rose AS, De Fabritiis G. DeepSite: Protein-binding site predictor using 3D-convolutional neural networks. Bioinformatics. 2017;**33**(19):3036-3042

[34] Kandel J, Tayara H, Chong KT. PUResNet: Prediction of protein-ligand binding sites using deep residual neural network. Journal of Cheminformatics. 2021;**13**(1):65

[35] Huang SY, Zou X. Advances and Challenges in Protein-Ligand Docking. IJMS. 2010;**11**(8):3016-3034

[36] de Vries SJ, van Dijk M, Bonvin AMJJ. The HADDOCK web server for data-driven biomolecular docking. Nature Protocols. 2010;**5**(5):883-897

[37] Fan J, Fu A, Zhang L. Progress in molecular docking. Quantitative Biology. 2019;**7**(2):83-89

[38] Crampon K, Giorkallos A, Deldossi M, Baud S, Steffenel LA. Machine-learning methods for ligand–protein molecular docking. Drug Discovery Today. 2022;**27**(1):151-164

[39] Jiang F, Kim SH. "Soft docking": Matching of molecular surface cubes. Journal of Molecular Biology. 1991;**219**(1):79-102

[40] Ferrari AM, Wei BQ, Costantino L, Shoichet BK. Soft docking and multiple receptor conformations in virtual screening. Journal of Medicinal Chemistry. 2004;**47**(21):5076-5084

[41] Torres PHM, Sodero ACR, Jofily P, Silva-Jr FP. Key topics in molecular docking for drug design. IJMS. 2019;**20**(18):4574

[42] Gioia D, Bertazzo M, Recanatini M, Masetti M, Cavalli A. Dynamic docking: A paradigm shift in computational drug discovery. Molecules. 2017;**22**(11):2029

[43] Sousa SF, Fernandes PA, Ramos MJ. Protein-ligand docking: Current status and future challenges. Proteins. 2006;**65**(1):15-26

[44] Meng XY, Zhang HX, Mezei M, Cui M. Molecular docking: A powerful approach for structure-based drug discovery. Caduceus. 2011;**7**(2):146-157

[45] Kuntz ID, Blaney JM, Oatley SJ, Langridge R, Ferrin TE. A geometric approach to macromolecule-ligand interactions. Journal of Molecular Biology. 1982;**161**(2):269-288

[46] Miller MD, Kearsley SK, Underwood DJ, Sheridan RP. FLOG: A system to select ?quasi-flexible? ligands complementary to a receptor of known three-dimensional structure. Journal of Computer-Aided Molecular Design. 1994;**8**(2):153-174

[47] Pang YP, Perola E, Xu K, Prendergast FG. EUDOC: A computer program for identification of drug interaction sites in macromolecules and drug leads from chemical databases. Journal of Computational Chemistry. 2001;**22**(15):1750-1771

[48] Jain AN. Surflex: Fully automatic flexible molecular docking using a molecular similarity-based search engine. Journal of Medicinal Chemistry. 2003;**46**(4):499-511

[49] Diller DJ, Merz KM. High throughput docking for library design and library prioritization. Proteins. 2001;**43**(2):113-124

[50] Burkhard P, Taylor P, Walkinshaw MD. An example of a protein ligand found by database mining: Description of the docking method and its verification by a 2.3 Å X-ray structure of a Thrombin-Ligand complex. Journal of Molecular Biology. 1998;**277**(2):449-466

[51] Huang SY, Zou X. Ensemble docking of multiple protein structures: Considering protein structural variations in molecular docking. Proteins. 2006;**66**(2):399-421

[52] Prieto-Martínez FD, Arciniega M, Medina-Franco JL. Acoplamiento Molecular: Avances Recientes y Retos. TIP RECQB. 2018. [cited 2022 May 15];21. Available from: http://tip.

zaragoza.unam.mx/index.php/tip/article/view/143

[53] Guedes IA, de Magalhães CS, Dardenne LE. Receptor–ligand molecular docking. Biophysical Reviews. 2014;**6**(1):75-87

[54] Friesner RA, Banks JL, Murphy RB, Halgren TA, Klicic JJ, Mainz DT, et al. Glide: A new approach for rapid, accurate docking and scoring. 1. Method and assessment of docking accuracy. Journal of Medicinal Chemistry. 2004;**47**(7):1739-1749

[55] McGann MR, Almond HR, Nicholls A, Grant JA, Brown FK. Gaussian docking functions. Biopolymers. 2003;**68**(1):76-90

[56] Ewing TJA, Kuntz ID. Critical evaluation of search algorithms for automated molecular docking and database screening. Journal of Computational Chemistry. 1997;**18**(9):1175-1189

[57] Böhm HJ. The computer program LUDI: A new method for the de novo design of enzyme inhibitors. Journal of Computer-Aided Molecular Design. 1992;**6**(1):61-78

[58] Rarey M, Kramer B, Lengauer T, Klebe G. A fast flexible docking method using an incremental construction algorithm. Journal of Molecular Biology. 1996;**261**(3):470-489

[59] Bentham Science Publisher BSP. eHiTS: An innovative approach to the docking and scoring function problems. CPPS. 2006;7(5):421-435

[60] Trott O, Olson AJ. AutoDock Vina: Improving the speed and accuracy of docking with a new scoring function, efficient optimization, and multithreading. Journal of Computational Chemistry. 2009

[61] Verdonk ML, Cole JC, Hartshorn MJ, Murray CW, Taylor RD. Improved protein-ligand docking using GOLD. Proteins. 2003;**52**(4):609-623

[62] de Magalhães CS, Almeida DM, Barbosa HJC, Dardenne LE. A dynamic niching genetic algorithm strategy for docking highly flexible ligands. Information Sciences. 2014;**289**:206-224

[63] Thomsen R, Christensen MH. MolDock: A new technique for high-accuracy molecular docking. Journal of Medicinal Chemistry. 2006;**49**(11):3315-3321

[64] Forli S, Huey R, Pique ME, Sanner MF, Goodsell DS, Olson AJ. Computational protein–ligand docking and virtual drug screening with the AutoDock suite. Nature Protocols. 2016;**11**(5):905-919

[65] Bentham Science Publisher BSP. Scoring functions for protein-ligand docking. CPPS. 2006;**7**(5):407-420

[66] Weiner PK, Kollman PA. AMBER: Assisted model building with energy refinement. A general program for modeling molecules and their interactions. Journal of Computational Chemistry. 1981;**2**(3):287-303

[67] Brooks BR, Bruccoleri RE, Olafson BD, States DJ, Swaminathan S, Karplus M. CHARMM: A program for macromolecular energy, minimization, and dynamics calculations. Journal of Computational Chemistry. 1983;**4**(2):187-217

[68] van Gunsteren WF, Berendsen HJC. Computer simulation of molecular dynamics: Methodology, applications, and perspectives in chemistry. Angewandte Chemie (International Ed. in English). 1990;**29**(9):992-1023

[69] Jorgensen WL, Tirado-Rives J. The OPLS Potential Functions for Proteins. Energy Minimizations for Crystals of Cyclic Peptides and Crambin. p. 10

[70] Parrill AL, Reddy MR. Rational Drug Design: Novel Methodology and Practical Applications. American Chemical Society; 1999 [cited 2022 May 23]. (ACS Symposium Series; vol. 719). Available from: https://pubs.acs.org/doi/book/10.1021/bk-1999-0719

[71] Krammer A, Kirchhoff PD, Jiang X, Venkatachalam CM, Waldman M. LigScore: A novel scoring function for predicting binding affinities. Journal of Molecular Graphics & Modelling. 2005;**23**(5):395-407

[72] Böhm HJ. The development of a simple empirical scoring function to estimate the binding constant for a protein-ligand complex of known three-dimensional structure. Journal of Computer-Aided Molecular Design. 1994;**8**(3):243-256

[73] Wang R, Liu L, Lai L, Tang Y. SCORE: A new empirical method for estimating the binding affinity of a protein-ligand complex. Journal of Molecular Modeling. 1998;**4**(12):379-394

[74] Wang R, Lai L, Wang S. Further development and validation of empirical scoring functions for structure-based binding affinity prediction. Journal of Computer-Aided Molecular Design. 2002;**16**(1):11-26

[75] Dias R, de Azevedo W. Molecular docking algorithms. CDT. 2008;**9**(12):1040-1047

[76] Waszkowycz B, Clark DE, Gancia E. Outstanding challenges in protein–ligand docking and structure-based virtual screening. WIREs Computational Molecular Science. 2011;**1**(2):229-259

[77] Morris GM, Lim-Wilby M. Molecular docking. In: Kukol A, editor. Molecular Modeling of Proteins. Totowa, NJ: Humana Press; 2008. pp. 365-382

[78] Verdonk ML, Taylor RD, Chessari G, Murray CW. Illustration of current challenges in molecular docking. In: Structure-Based Drug Discovery. Dordrecht: Springer Netherlands; 2007. pp. 201-221

[79] Janin J, Henrick K, Moult J, Eyck LT, Sternberg MJE, Vajda S, et al. CAPRI: A critical assessment of PRedicted interactions. Proteins. 2003;**52**(1):2-9

[80] Janin J. Protein–protein docking tested in blind predictions: The CAPRI experiment. Molecular BioSystems. 2010;**6**(12):2351

[81] Hurle MR, Yang L, Xie Q, Rajpal DK, Sanseau P, Agarwal P. Computational drug repositioning: From data to therapeutics. Clinical Pharmacology and Therapeutics. 2013;**93**(4):335-341

[82] Scherman D, Fetro C. Drug repositioning for rare diseases: Knowledge-based success stories. Thérapie. 2020;**75**(2):161-167

[83] Xiao H, Bid HK, Chen X, Wu X, Wei J, Bian Y, et al. Repositioning Bazedoxifene as a novel IL-6/GP130 signaling antagonist for human rhabdomyosarcoma therapy. PLoS ONE. 2017;**12**(7):e0180297

[84] Gupta RR. Application of artificial intelligence and machine learning in drug discovery. Methods in Molecular Biology. 2022;**2390**:113-124

[85] Thomas M, Boardman A, Garcia-Ortegon M, Yang H, de Graaf C, Bender A. Applications of artificial intelligence in drug design: Opportunities and challenges. Methods in Molecular Biology. 2022;**2390**:1-59

[86] Zhu T, Cao S, Su PC, Patel R, Shah D, Chokshi HB, et al. Hit identification and optimization in virtual screening: Practical recommendations based on a critical literature analysis: Miniperspective. Journal of Medicinal Chemistry. 2013;**56**(17):6560-6572

[87] Neves BJ, Mottin M, Moreira-Filho JT, Sousa BK de P, Mendonca SS, Andrade CH. Best practices for docking-based virtual screening. In: Molecular Docking for Computer-Aided Drug Design. Academic Press (Elsevier); 2021. pp. 75-98

[88] Lipinski CA, Lombardo F, Dominy BW, Feeney PJ. Experimental and computational approaches to estimate solubility and permeability in drug discovery and development settings. Advanced Drug Delivery Reviews. 2001;**46**(1-3):3-26

[89] Veber DF, Johnson SR, Cheng HY, Smith BR, Ward KW, Kopple KD. Molecular properties that influence the oral bioavailability of drug candidates. Journal of Medicinal Chemistry. 2002;**45**(12):2615-2623

[90] Neves BJ, Braga RC, Melo-Filho CC, Moreira-Filho JT, Muratov EN, Andrade CH. QSAR-based virtual screening: Advances and applications in drug discovery. Frontiers in Pharmacology. 2018;**9**:1275

[91] Fassio AV, Santos LH, Silveira SA, Ferreira RS, de Melo-Minardi RC. nAPOLI: A graph-based strategy to detect and visualize conserved protein-ligand interactions in large-scale. IEEE/ACM Transactions on Computational Biology and Bioinformatics. 2019:1-1

[92] Kurogi Y, Güner OF. Pharmacophore modeling and three-dimensional database searching for drug design using catalyst. Current Medicinal Chemistry. 2001;**8**(9):1035-1055

[93] Dixon SL, Smondyrev AM, Knoll EH, Rao SN, Shaw DE, Friesner RA. PHASE: A new engine for pharmacophore perception, 3D QSAR model development, and 3D database screening: 1. Methodology and preliminary results. Journal of Computer-Aided Molecular Design. 2006;**20**(10-11):647-671

[94] Chen X, Rusinko A, Tropsha A, Young SS. Automated pharmacophore identification for large chemical data sets. Journal of Chemical Information and Computer Sciences. 1999;**39**(5):887-896

[95] Schneidman-Duhovny D, Dror O, Inbar Y, Nussinov R, Wolfson HJ. PharmaGist: A webserver for ligand-based pharmacophore detection. Nucleic Acids Research. 2008;**36**:W223-W228

[96] Fan N, Bauer CA, Stork C, de Bruyn KC, Kirchmair J. ALADDIN: Docking approach augmented by machine learning for protein structure selection yields superior virtual screening performance. Molecular Informatics. 2020;**39**(4):e1900103

[97] Rashidieh B, Molakarimi M, Mohseni A, Tria SM, Truong H, Srihari S, et al. Targeting BRF2 in cancer using repurposed drugs. Cancers. 2021;**13**(15):3778

[98] Berman HM. The protein data bank. Nucleic Acids Research. 2000;**28**(1):235-242

[99] Chen X. TTD: Therapeutic target database. Nucleic Acids Research. 2002;**30**(1):412-415

[100] Chen YZ, Zhi DG. Ligand-protein inverse docking and its potential use in the computer search of protein targets of a small molecule. Proteins. 2001;**43**(2):217-226

[101] Wang JC, Chu PY, Chen CM, Lin JH. idTarget: A web server for identifying protein targets of small chemical molecules with robust scoring functions and a divide-and-conquer docking approach. Nucleic Acids Research. 2012;**40**:W393-W399

[102] Xie T, Zhang L, Zhang S, Ouyang L, Cai H, Liu B. ACTP: A webserver for predicting potential targets and relevant pathways of autophagy-modulating compounds. Oncotarget. 2016;**7**(9):10015-10022

[103] Lee A, Kim D. CRDS: Consensus reverse docking system for target fishing. Bioinformatics. 2019

[104] Stepanova EE, Balandina SY, Drobkova VA, Dmitriev MV, Mashevskaya IV, Maslivets AN. Synthesis, in vitro antibacterial activity against *Mycobacterium tuberculosis*, and reverse docking-based target fishing of 1,4-benzoxazin-2-one derivatives. Archiv der Pharmazie. 2021;**354**(2):2000199

[105] Imrie F, Bradley AR, van der Schaar M, Deane CM. Protein family-specific models using deep neural networks and transfer learning improve virtual screening and highlight the need for more data. Journal of Chemical Information and Modeling. 2018;**58**(11):2319-2330

[106] Kitchen DB, Decornez H, Furr JR, Bajorath J. Docking and scoring in virtual screening for drug discovery: Methods and applications. Nature Reviews. Drug Discovery. 2004;**3**(11):935-949

[107] Yuan S, Chan HCS, Hu Z. Using PyMOL as a platform for computational drug design. WIREs Computers Molecular Science. 2017;**30**(2):70

[108] Koukos PI, Réau M, Bonvin AMJJ. Shape-restrained modeling of protein–small-molecule complexes with high ambiguity driven DOCKing. Journal of Chemical Information and Modeling. 2021;**61**(9):4807-4818

[109] Koukos PI, Xue LC, Bonvin AMJJ. Protein–ligand pose and affinity prediction: Lessons from D3R Grand Challenge 3. Journal of Computer-Aided Molecular Design. 2019;**33**(1):83-91

[110] Stanzione F, Giangreco I, Cole JC. Use of molecular docking computational tools in drug discovery. In: Progress in Medicinal Chemistry. Elsevier; 2021. pp. 273-343

[111] Sennhauser G, Amstutz P, Briand C, Storchenegger O, Grütter MG. Drug export pathway of multidrug exporter AcrB revealed by DARPin inhibitors. PLoS Biology. 2007;**5**(1):e7

[112] Grosdidier A, Zoete V, Michielin O. SwissDock, a protein-small molecule docking web service based on EADock DSS. Nucleic Acids Research. 2011;**39**(suppl):W270-W277

[113] Guex N, Peitsch MC. SWISS-MODEL and the Swiss-Pdb Viewer: An environment for comparative protein modeling. Electrophoresis. 1997;**18**(15):2714-2723

Chapter 3

Molecular Docking: Metamorphosis in Drug Discovery

Kishor Danao, Deweshri Nandurkar, Vijayshri Rokde, Ruchi Shivhare and Ujwala Mahajan

Abstract

Molecular docking is recognized a part of computer-aided drug design that is mostly used in medicinal chemistry. It has proven to be an effective, quick, and low-cost technique in both scientific and corporate contexts. It helps in rationalizing the ligands activity towards a target to perform structure-based drug design (SBDD). Docking assists the revealing of novel compound of therapeutic interest, forecasting ligand-protein interaction at a molecular basis and delineating structure activity relationships (SARs). Molecular docking acts as a boon to identify promising agents in emergence of diseases which endangering the human health. In this chapter, we engrossed on the techniques, types, opportunities, challenges and success stories of molecular docking in drug development.

Keywords: molecular docking, drug discovery, ligand-protein interaction, SAR, molecular recognition, drug design

1. Introduction

Medicinal chemistry relates to the design and production of compounds that can be used in medicine for the prevention, treatment or cure of human and animal diseases. Medicinal chemistry includes the study of existing drugs for their biological properties and structure activity relationships (SARs) [1, 2]. The discovery and development of a new drug with desired therapeutic activity is a long, tedious and expensive process. The industry statistics suggest that up to 10,000 compounds are synthesized and tested, up to 100 compounds are assessed for safety and only 10 compounds are tested clinically in humans for every drug that is approved for medical use. Today it takes approximately ten years and requires high cost to bring a new drug in market. In spite of the tremendous costs involved the payoff is also high and improvement made in preventing and controlling human disease. Even when the new drugs come in the market its success is not assured [3, 4]. Many centuries ago, human beings started using chemicals to treat the diseases. Hippocrates recommended the use of metallic salts such as copper and zinc, iron sulphate and cadmium oxide as drugs. In 1500 A.D., Carpensis employed mercuric compounds to treat syphilis. Urea was the first organic compounds to be synthesized in laboratory by Wohler in 1852. Between eighteenth and nineteenth century, several organic compounds were synthesized which included drugs such as salicylic acid (Kolbe), antipyrine (Knorr), aspirin (Dresser), barbital (Emil Fischer and Mering), prontosil, the first sulpha drug (G. Domagk), chlorpromazine (Charpentier), phenyl magnesium bromide (Victor Grignard), polyethers (Charles J. Pedersen) and others [5]. Except, the therapeutic utility of these agents, nothing more was known about their mechanism of action and it was only believed that they were effective because of their physicochemical parameters like partition coefficient, hydrogen bonding, van der Waal's forces, dipole-dipole interactions and anionic bonds, etc. [6, 7]. Earlier to the chemical era, it was the natural products mostly from plant sources, which were used in therapeutics. Later, progress in knowledge of chemistry helped to isolate and identify the active ingredients in plants. Some of the outstanding achievements of such phytochemical approach include the discoveries such as digitalis glycosides from foxglove plant by William Withering in 1785; the opium alkaloids like morphine and codeine from poppy plant by Serturner in 1806; anti-malarial such as quinine, quinidine, cinchonine from cinchona bark by Pelletier and Dumas in 1823; belladonna alkaloids like atropine and scopolamine by Mein in 1833; rauwolfia alkaloids (reserpine and deserpidine) by Muller et al. in 1952, etc. In addition, many important natural products like antibiotics, steroids and peptide hormones, vitamins, enzymes, prostaglandins and pheromones were discovered in the concurrent period [8, 9]. The synthesis of compounds is followed by screening of its pharmacological actions. The observation of interest and repeatable biological activity in such screening had always opened the pathways for additional chemical research to prepare their analogs so as to obtain significant newer medicinal products. A small change in structure frequently leads a profound change in the pharmacological effect. This logic has prompted to synthesize derivatives of natural compounds and the structural analogues of biologically interesting substances with the "lead" (prototype) compound [10]. Many of the currently used antispasmodics [11–14] (dicyclomine, cyclopentolate, clidinium bromide, mebeverine, metoclopramide, tropicamide), antibiotics [15–20] (penicillins, cloxacillin, amoxacillin, ampicillin, cefadroxil, cefaclor, cefixime, cefepime), sulphonamides [21–25] (sulphacetamide, sulphadiazine, sulphasalazine, sulphamethoxazole), anthelmintics [26–28] (albendazole, mebedazole, pyrantel pamoate, piperazine, diethylcarbamazine citrate, praziquantel, niclosamide), antimycobacterials [29–31] (clofazimine, dapsone, ethambutol, isoniazid, benzothiazole, sulphonamide, rifampin), analgesics [32–35] (aspirin, diclofenac sodium, ibuprofen, indomethacin, ketoprofen, naproxen, piroxicam), anticonvulsants [36–40] (phenytoin, ethosuximide, carbamazepine, sodium valproate, riluzole), antitumours [41–46] (amsacrine, azacitidine, chlorambucil, cyclosporine, fluorouracil), diuretics [47–51] (acetazolamide, chlorothiazide, furosemide, triamterene, spironolactone), antimalarials [52–56] (chloroquine, primaquine, amodiaquine, proguanil, pyrimethamine), antifungals [57–60] (griseofulvin, nystatin, miconazole, tolnaftate, clotrimazole), antihistaminics [61–65] (chlorpheniramine maleate, promethazine, astemizole, cetirizine hydro-chloride, fexofenadine) have been obtained by synthetic or semi-synthetic approach. In recent years, the molecular studies are more directed to discover new targets for better treatment of the disease. In addition, newer screening methods of assays, studying the effect of drug on the cell lines, availability of purified or recombinant enzymes and improved understanding about the nature and properties of receptor systems immensely boosted the drug research. It is well recognized that a medicinal chemist had been a key person in the discovery of a new drug. He synthesizes a new drug, isolates and characterizes natural products and in association of pharmacologist establishes a rational SAR. Moreover, SAR had proved to be vital and fundamental to drug discovery [66].

1.1 Discovery of drugs of the future

Traditionally, new medications have been discovered by screening a large number of synthetic chemical compounds or natural items for desired effects. Although this method of developing novel pharmacological agents has proven to be successful in the past, it is not optimal for a variety of reasons. The most significant disadvantage of the screening approach is the demand for a proper screening procedure. Another problem with the screening process is that because of its random nature, it is inherently repetitious and time consuming just to find a chemical with the desired activity [67, 68]. Drugs can be created particularly to interact with the target molecule in such a way that the disease is disrupted after the disease process is understood at the molecular level and the target molecule (s) is defined. Because of the large quantity of data that must be gathered in order to produce medications using this method, here is where computer-aided drug design will have the most influence [69, 70].

In discussing various techniques of finding new drugs described in **Figure 1**, it is important to remember that drug discovery is both a cumulative and a reiterative process. Drugs developed mechanistically will likely to be screened and later modified in order to produce the best candidate design [71]. The use of stiff constructs for structure and targets is common in the early stages of using molecular modelling to create medications. In medication design, the flexibility of molecular information, both in single molecules and in molecules interacting with each other, is a crucial and difficult subject.

Since, the discovery of morphine in 1806 lot many important drugs came for remedy of humans, important results in drug discovery during last three centuries is shown in **Table 1**.

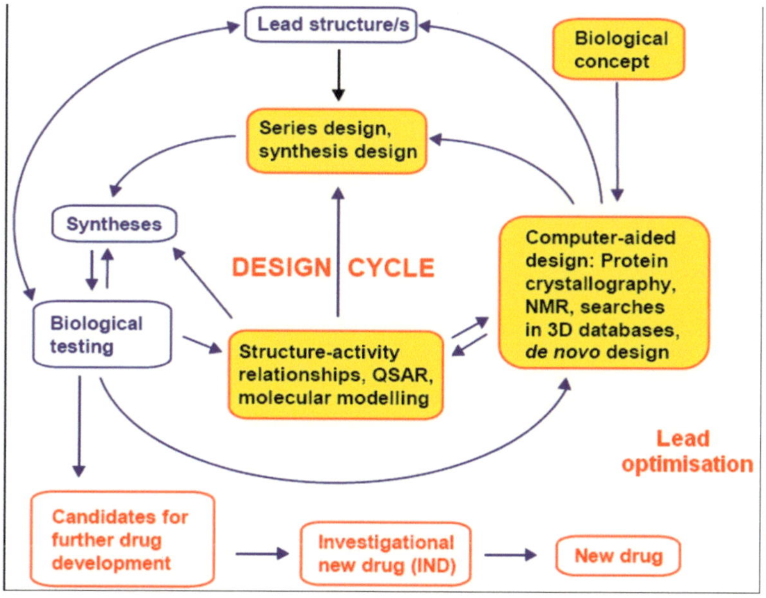

Figure 1.
Lead optimization cycle.

Year	Drug	Biological action	Year	Drug	Biological action
1806	Morphine	Hypnotic agent	1990	Ondansetron	Antiemetic agent (5-HT3 blocker)
1875	Salicylic acid	Anti-inflammatory agent	1991	Sumatriptan	Anti-migraine agent (5-HT1 blocker)
1884	Cocaine	Stimulant, local anaesthetic agent	1993	Risperidon	Antipsychotic agent (D2/5-HT2 blocker)
1888	Phenacetin	Analgesic and antipyretic agent	1994	Famciclovir	Anti-herpes (DNA polymerase inhibitor)
1899	Acetylsalicylic acid	Analgesic and antipyretic agent	1995	Losartan	Antihypertensive agent (A II antagonist)
1903	Barbiturates	Sedatives	1995	Dorzolamide	Glaucoma (carbonic anhydrase inhibit.)
1909	Arsphenamine	Antisyphilitic agent	1996	Nevirapin	HIV reverse transcriptase inhibitor
1921	Procaine	Local anaesthetic agent	1996	Indinavir, Ritonavir,	HIV protease inhibitors
1922	Insulin	Antidiabetic agent	1997	Saquinavir	HIV protease inhibitor
1928	Estrone	Female sex hormone	1997	Finasteride	Hair loss
1928	Penicillin	Antibiotic agent	1998	Sibutramine	Adipositas (lipase inhibitor)
1935	Sulphachrysoidine	Bacteriostatic agent	1998	Orlistat	Adipositas (lipase inhibitor)
1944	Streptomycin	Antibiotic agent	1999	Sildenafil	Erectile dysfunction
1945	Chloroquine	Antimalarial agent	2000	Celecoxib, Rofecoxib	Anti-arthritis agents (COX-2 inhibitors)
1952	Chlorpromazine	Neuroleptic agent	2001	Amprenavir	HIV protease inhibitor
1956	Tolbutamide	Oral antidiabetic agent	2002	Cyclosporine A	Thrombosis (synthetic LMWH)
1960	Chlordiazepoxide	Tranquillizer	2002	Imantinib	CML (specific ABL-TK inhibitor)
1962	Verapamil	Calcium channel blocker	2005	Telmesetan	Potassium pump inhibitor
1963	Propranolol	Antihypertensive agent (beta-blocker)	2007	Oseltamavir	Antiviral
1964	Furosemide	Diuretic agent	2008	Saxgliptin	Antidiabetic (DPP-4 inhibitor)
1971	L-dopa	Anti-Parkinson agent	2010	Fingolimod	Multiple sclerosis
1975	Nifedipine	Calcium channel blocker	2012	Avanafil	Erective dysfunction
1976	Cimetidine	Anti-ulcers agent (H2 blocker)	2013	Riociguat	Hypertension
1981	Captopril	Antihypertensive agent (ACE inhibitor)	2014	Dapagliflozin	Type II diabetes
1981	Ranitidine	Anti-ulcers agent (H2 blocker)	2015	Ivabradin	Heart failure
1983	Cyclosporine A	Immunosuppressant	2016	Rucaparib	Ovarian cancer

Year	Drug	Biological action	Year	Drug	Biological action
1984	Enalapril	Antihypertensive agent (ACE inhibitor)	2017	Plecanatide	Chronic constipation
1985	Mefloquine	Antimalarial agent	2018	Annovera	Contraceptive
1986	Fluoxetine	Antidepressant (5-HT transporter)	2019	Ubrogepant	Migrain
1987	Artemisinin	Antimalarial agent	2021	Pafolacianine	Cancer
1988	Omeprazole	Anti-ulcer agent (H/K-ATPase inhibitor)	2022	Pafolacianine	Insomnia

Table 1.
Important results in drug discovery.

1.2 Computer-aided drug design

Drug research and discovery is a time-consuming and costly procedure. In order to get a medicine to market, it takes an average of 10–15 years and $500–800 million dollars [72]. This is why, in order to speed up the process, computer-assisted drug design (CADD) technologies have become popular in the pharmaceutical business. CADD, as shown in **Figure 2**, assists scientists in focusing on the most promising compounds in order to reduce the amount of time and money spent on synthetic and biological testing.

In reality, the availability of experimentally defined 3D (three-dimensional) structures of target proteins usually determines which CADD techniques are used. If the structure of a protein is unknown, ligand-based drug design methods such as quantitative structure activity relationship (QSAR) and pharmacophore analysis can be used. If the target structures are known, structure-based techniques such as molecular docking can be utilised to create novel active molecules with improved potency using the target 3D structures. The accuracy of prediction is anticipated to improve as more structures become accessible. In the absence of the receptor 3D information, lead identification and optimization depend on available pharmacologically relevant agents and their bioactivities [73, 74]. The computational approaches include QSAR, pharmacophore modelling and database mining. QSAR can be taken as an example to

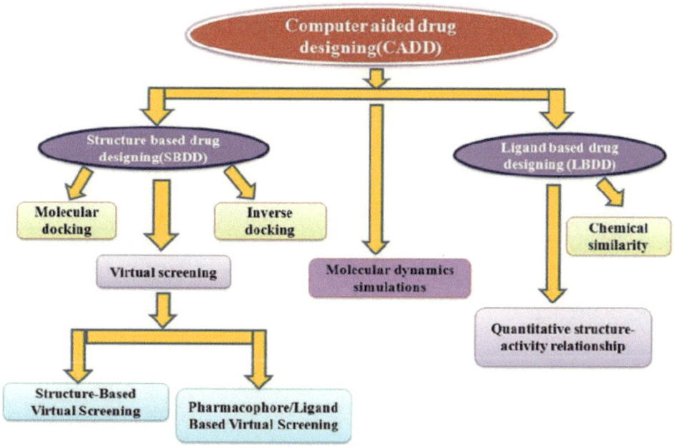

Figure 2.
Computer-aided drug design.

illustrate the workflow. A mathematical relationship between structural features and target properties of a group of compounds is described by QSAR. Over the last few decades, many various 2D (two-dimensional) and 3D QSAR techniques have been developed [75]. Chemical descriptors and mathematical procedures used to build the association between the goal attributes and the descriptors are two key differences between these strategies.

Many graph theoretic indices-based 2D QSAR algorithms have been thoroughly researched. Although the physical significance of these indices is unknown, they do indicate various characteristics of molecular structures. It's been used to predict biological activity in analytical chemistry, toxicology analysis, and other fields. To overcome the shortcomings of 2D QSAR techniques, such as their inability to differentiate stereoisomers, 3D QSAR approaches have been developed. Molecular shape analysis (MSA), distance geometry, and Voronoi procedures are examples of 3D methodologies. The most well-known example of 3D QSAR is comparative molecular field analysis (CoMFA). By elegantly merging the power of molecular graphics and the partial least square (PLS) technique, it has been widely employed in medicinal chemistry and toxicity studies. The linear relationship between a target property and molecular descriptors is frequently assumed in QSAR approaches. However, the rapid development of structural and biological data has put this assumption to the test. To this goal, a number of nonlinear QSAR algorithms have been presented, the majority of which are based on artificial neural network (ANN) or machine learning techniques [76]. Scientists had always concentrated on the development and application of automated algorithms for QSAR studies, including genetic algorithms (GAs)-partial least squares, k-nearest neighbour (k-NN), and support vector machine (SVM). Learning approaches have been widely used in cheminformatics and molecular modelling. For instance, SVM was found to yield better results compared to multiple linear regressions (MLR) and radial basis functions (RBF).

SBDD (structure-based drug design) has played a significant role in drug development and discovery [76]. Understanding receptor–ligand interactions is required for this strategy. The target 3D structure can be used to develop new ligands if it is known. X-ray crystallography, NMR, and homology modelling are all used to obtain structural information. SBDD methods are used to assess complementarities and anticipate potential binding modes and affinities between small compounds and their macromolecular receptors. SBDD's success is extensively proven, and computational approaches differ greatly in methodology, performance, and speed. Some can provide accurate binding modes, while others are better suited to scanning vast datasets quickly [77].

2. Molecular docking study

The production, manipulation, or representation of 3D structures of molecules and their associated physicochemical properties is referred to as molecular docking. It entails a variety of computational strategies for predicting chemical and biological properties based on theoretical chemistry methodologies and experimental data. The subject is sometimes referred to as "molecular graphics," "molecular visualisations," "computational chemistry," or "computational quantum chemistry," depending on the context and rigour. The molecular docking techniques are based on Huckel and Mullikan's conceptions of molecular orbitals and Westheimer et al. classical's mechanical programming.' The foundation of SBDD is 3D molecular structure [78, 79].

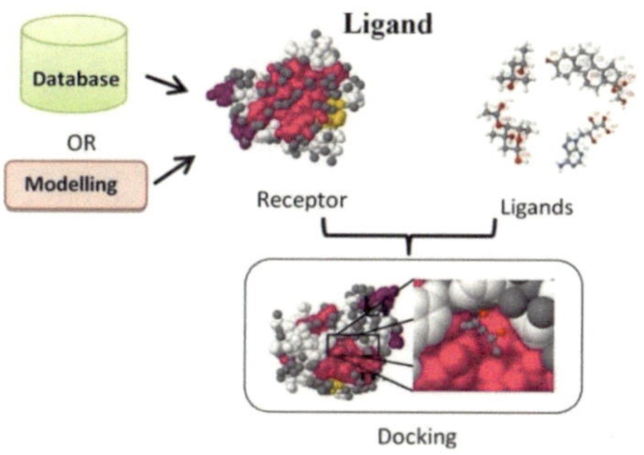

Figure 3.
Molecular docking process.

Separate data for protein structure and medication data are available, but no correlated data is accessible. Docking is the process of fitting two molecules together in complimentary styles in 3D space and designing the molecules rationally, as seen in **Figure 3**. Modeling a drug's interaction with its receptor is a difficult task. Hydrophobic, dispersion or van der Waals, hydrogen bonding, and electrostatic forces all play a role in intermolecular interaction. Hydrophobic interactions appear to be the dominant force for binding, whereas hydrogen bonding and electrostatic interactions appear to influence the specificity of the binding [80, 81].

2.1 Theory of docking

The objectives of molecular docking is to forecasting the ligand-receptor complex by using computer method. Docking is partitioned into two steps that is sampling ligand and scoring function. Sampling algorithms aid to find the energetically most favorable conformations of the ligand in the active site of the protein with their binding mode and further ranked these conformations using a scoring function.

2.1.1 Sampling algorithms

There are a great number of potential binding modes between two molecules due to the six degrees of translational and rotational freedom as well as the conformational degrees of freedom of both the ligand and protein [82]. Unfortunately, computing all of the conceivable conformations would be too expensive. In molecular docking software, various sampling techniques have been developed and are frequently utilized. In terms of shape features and chemical information, matching algorithms (MAs) based on molecular shape map a ligand onto an active site of a protein [83]. Pharmacophores represent the protein and the ligand. Each pharmacophore distance within the protein and ligand is determined for a match; the distance matrix between the pharmacophore and the associated ligand atoms governs new ligand conformations. During the match, chemical parameters such as hydrogen-bond donors and acceptors might be considered. Because MAs are fast, they can be used to enrich active chemicals from vast libraries. DOCK, FLOG, LibDock and SANDOCK programme provides ligand docking MAs [84–86]. The ligand is placed in an active site in a fragmented and incremental manner using incremental construction methods (ICMs). By breaking the ligands rotatable links, it is separated into many fragments, one of which is chosen to dock into the active site first. This anchor is typically the biggest fragment or the piece that has a functional purpose or interacts with protein. The remaining pieces can be added in stages. The ligand's flexibility is realized by generating different orientations to fit in the active site. DOCK 4.0, FlexX and SLIDE all use the ICM. In supplement to ICM, fragment-based approaches such as multiple copy simultaneous search (MCSS) and Ligue Universitaire D' Improvisation (LUDI) are used to create new ligands and modify existing ligands to improve their binding to the target protein. At the force field of the protein, MCSS creates 1000–5000 copies of a substituent, which are randomly put in the binding site of interest and subjected to simultaneous energy minimization and/or quenched molecular dynamics. Copies solely interact with proteins; interactions between copies are not included. Based on the interaction energies, a collection of energetically favorable binding sites and orientations for the functional group is discovered. Different functional categories are used to map the binding site. The linking of those different functional groups can be used to create new molecules that perfectly match the binding site [87]. The hydrogen bonds and hydrophobic interactions that potentially occur between the ligand and protein are the focus of LUDI. Interaction sites, which are discrete positions in space appropriate for establishing hydrogen bonds or filling a hydrophobic pocket, are the core notion. Using the rules or scanning the database, a set of interaction sites is constructed. After that, the fragment is fitted onto the interaction sites and distance criteria are used to evaluate it. The merging of some or all of the fitted fragments to a single molecule is the final stage. By randomly changing a ligand conformation or a population of ligands, stochastic methods seek the conformational space. Another well-known class of stochastic approaches is genetic algorithm (GA). The GA was inspired by Darwin's theory of evolution. The ligand's degrees of freedom are represented as binary strings called genes. These genes make up the "chromosome," which indicates the ligand's position. In GA, there are two types of genetic operators: mutation and crossover. Crossover swaps genes between two chromosomes, while mutation produces random changes to the genes. A novel ligand structure is created when genetic operators impact genes. New structures will be evaluated using a scoring system, and those that survive will be employed in the upcoming generation. AutoDock, GOLD, DIVALI, and DARWIN all use GAs [88–91].

2.1.2 Scoring functions

The scoring function's goal is to distinguish between proper and inappropriate poses, or binders and inactive substances, in a very short time. Scoring functions, on the other hand, require guessing rather than computing the protein-ligand binding affinity and through these functions, numerous assumptions and simplifications are used. There are three types of scoring functions: force-field-based, empirical, and knowledge-based. Basic force-field-based scoring functions calculate the sum of non-bonded (electrostatics and van der Waals) interactions to determine the binding energy. A Columbic framework is used to determine the electrostatic terms. Due to the difficulty of representing the protein's true environment with point charge calculations, a distance-dependent dielectric function is commonly utilized to regulate the contribution of charge–charge interactions [92–94]. A Lennard-Jones potential function describes the van der Waals terms. The "hardness" of the potential, which regulates how close a contact between protein and ligand atoms can be tolerated, can be varied by using different parameter sets for the Lennard-Jones potential. The processing speed of force-field-based scoring functions is also an issue. To address non-bonded interactions, cut-off distance is used. As a result, the accuracy of long-range effects involved in binding is reduced. Hydrogen bonds, solvations, and entropy contributions are considered in extensions of force-field-based scoring functions. DOCK, GOLD, and AutoDock are examples of software applications that provide these features [95]. They differ in their treatment of hydrogen bonding, the structure of the energy functions and other aspects. Furthermore, the accuracy of estimating binding energies can be improved by using other techniques also including linear interaction energy and free-energy perturbation methods (FEP) to refine the findings of docking with force-field-based functions. Binding energy is decomposed into multiple energy components in empirical scoring functions, including hydrogen bonds, ionic interactions, hydrophobic effect, and binding entropy. To arrive at a final score, each component is multiplied by a coefficient and then added together. Regression analysis fitted to a test set of ligand-protein complexes with known binding affinities yields coefficients. The energy terms in empirical scoring functions are quite simple to evaluate the affinities. Beyond the training set, however, it is unknown how well they are suited for ligand-protein complexes. Furthermore, various software may treat each term in empirical scoring functions differently, and the amount of terms included may differ as well. Examples of empirical scoring functions include LUDI, piecewise linear potential (PLP), and ChemScore. The interatomic interaction frequencies and/or distances between the ligand and protein are calculated using statistical analysis of ligand-protein complex crystal structures. They are founded on the notion that the more beneficial an encounter is, the more likely it will occur [96, 97]. Pairwise atom-type potentials are created from these frequency distributions. Within a particular cutoff, the score is derived by prioritizing favorable contacts and penalizing repulsive interactions between each atom in the ligand and protein. Knowledge-based functions are appealing because of their computational simplicity, which can be used to screen enormous compound datasets. They can also represent some unusual interactions, such as sulphur-aromatic or cation- that are frequently overlooked in empirical approaches. However, some interactions are underrepresented in the limited training sets of crystal structures, and the bias inherent in the selection of proteins for successful structure determination, so the obtained parameters may not be suitable for widespread use, particularly with implicating metals or halogens. knowledge-based functions such as DrugScore, SMoG, and Bleep that differ mostly in training set size, energy function shape, atom type definition, distance cutoff, and other characteristics [98–100]. Consensus scoring is a new technique for assessing docking conformation that combines numerous different scores. When a ligand or possible binder poses well in a number of different scoring schemes, it may be accepted. In virtual screening, consensus scoring usually enhances enrichment and improves the prediction of bound conformations and poses. However, binding energies predictions may still be wrong. When terms in distinct scoring functions are substantially connected, the utility of consensus scoring decreases. DOCK, ChemScore, PMF, GOLD, and FlexX scoring functions are all combined in CScore [101–103].

2.2 Docking methodologies

2.2.1 Docking of rigid ligand and rigid receptor

The search space is highly constrained when the ligand and receptor are both considered as rigid entities, with only three translational and three rotational degrees of freedom. In this scenario, ligand flexibility might be addressed by allowing for a degree of atom–atom overlap between the protein and the ligand, or by using a precomputed set of ligand conformations. Early versions of DOCK, FLOG, and certain protein-protein docking systems like FTDOCK used a mechanism that kept the ligand and receptor stiff during the docking process [104, 105].

DOCK is the world's initial automated process for docking a molecule into a receptor site, and it's still evolving. The ligand and receptor are represented as sets of spheres that can be superimposed using a clique detection approach. The ligand-receptor complexes are scored using geometrical and chemical MAs, and steric fit, chemical complementation, and pharmacophore similarity are all taken into account. To account for ligand flexibility, incremental construction approach and exhaustive search have been included to the enhanced versions.

The extensive search generates a user-defined number of conformers at random, which is a multiple of the ligand's rotatable bonds. In terms of scoring, DOCK 6.4 now includes AMBER derived forcefield scoring with implicit solvent. Also, the molecular mechanics methodologies such as Poisson–Boltzmann or generalized Born and surface area continuum solvation (MM/PBSA and MM/GBSA) methods are used to determine the chemisorption which estimate the free energy of the binding of small ligands to biological macromolecules [106].

FLOG creates ligand conformations based on distance geometry and calculates the sets of distances using a search technique. For some flexibility, up to 25 specified conformations of the ligand might be employed to dock. Users can identify critical sites that must be associated with ligand atoms using FLOG. If a critical interaction is already known before docking, this method is useful. Van der Waals, electrostatics, hydrogen bonding, and hydrophobic interactions are all taken into account when scoring conformations [107].

2.2.2 Docking of flexible ligand and rigid receptor

As both the ligand and the receptor change conformations to form a minimum energy perfect-fit complex in systems that follow the induced fit paradigm, it is critical to consider the flexibility of both the ligand and receptor. However, when the receptor is also flexible, the cost is very high. As a result, the most typical technique is to consider the ligand as flexible while keeping the receptor stiff during docking, which is likewise a trade-off between accuracy and computational time. Almost all docking applications, such as AutoDock and FlexX, have embraced this concept [108–110]. To mimic ligand flexibility while keeping the receptor stiff, AutoDock 3.0 uses Monte Carlo simulated annealing, evolutionary, genetic, and Lamarckian genetic algorithm (LGA) approaches. The AMBER force field, which includes van der Waals, hydrogen bonding, electrostatic interactions, conformational entropy, and desolvation components, is used to calculate the scoring function. An empirical scaling factor derived from experimental data is used to weight each term. By enabling side-chains to shift, AutoDock 4.0 can model receptor flexibility. In this version of AutoDock, you may also test the interaction of protein-protein docking [111–114]. The latest version of AutoDock Vina for molecular docking and virtual screening was recently published. By redocking the 190 receptor-ligand complexes that had been utilised as a training set for the AutoDock 4, AutoDock Vina demonstrated a two-order exponential increase in speed as well as a considerable improvement in binding mode prediction accuracy [115]. FlexX samples ligand conformations using an incremental building approach. By matching hydrogen bond pairings and metal and aromatic ring interactions between the ligand and protein, the base fragment is docked into the active site. The remaining components are then built up incrementally in line with a set of preset rotatable torsion angles to complete the structure. Electrostatic interactions, directional hydrogen bonds, rotational entropy, and aromatic and lipophilic interactions are all included in the present edition. The relationships between functional groups are also considered when group types and geometry are assigned [116].

2.2.3 Docking of flexible ligand and flexible receptor

In flexible docking, the docking of the ligand and receptor is difficult task due to protein intrinsic mobility and ligand binding affinity. MD simulations might theoretically model all degrees of freedom in the ligand-receptor combination. However, MD has the previously discussed issue of insufficient sampling. Another stumbling block is the method's high computing cost, which prevents it from being employed in large-scale chemical database screening [117]. Several theoretical models, including conformer selection and conformational induction, have been presented to illustrate the flexible ligand-protein binding process in addition to the historic induced fit. Conformer selection refers to a process in which a ligand selects a favourable conformation from a variety of protein conformations, while conformational induction describes a process in which the ligand induces the protein to adopt a conformation that it would not adopt spontaneously in its unbound state. This conformational change is sometimes compared to a partial refolding of the protein [118]. The most basic is "soft-docking," which lowers the van der Waals repulsion energy term in the scoring function to allow for some atom-to-atom overlap between the receptor and the ligand. This strategy could be lacking in versatility. Nonetheless, it has the advantage of computational efficiency because the receptor coordinates are fixed, and the van der Waals parameters are readily adjusted. To deal with side chain flexibility, AutoDock 4 uses a simultaneous sampling technique. Users can select multiple side chains of the receptor and sample them simultaneously with a ligand using the same methods. During sampling, other parts of the receptor are handled strictly using a grid energy map. Grid energy maps were established to hold receptor energy information and facilitate ligand-receptor interaction energy calculations [119]. Another approach to dealing with protein flexibility is to use an ensemble of protein conformations, which corresponds to conformer selection theory. Instead of docking into a single rigid protein conformation, a ligand is docked into a set of hard protein conformations and the results are merged using the method of choice. This method was first used in DOCK, which constructs an ensemble's average potential energy grid and has since been extended in a variety of programmes. Discrete protein conformations are sampled in a combinatorial approach during the gradual building of a ligand. Based on a comparison of the ligand and each alternative, the highest scoring protein structure is chosen (**Table 2**).

Because there are so many degrees of freedom and little knowledge of the effect of solvent on the binding relationship, modelling the intermolecular interactions in a ligand-protein complex is difficult. The docking of a ligand to a binding site attempts to emulate the natural course of interaction between the ligand and its receptor by taking the shortest path possible. Although there are straightforward ways for docking rigid ligands with rigid receptors and flexible ligands with rigid receptors, docking conformationally flexible ligands and receptors is more difficult. The interaction of macromolecular receptors and tiny drug molecules is a crucial stage in regulatory systems, drug pharmacology, hazardous side effects, and other processes.

The structure of protein-ligand or protein-protein binding sites is exploited in SBDD, however the site is not always known at the outset. Even if the site is identified, researchers may want to look for other potential binding sites that could lead to distinct biological effects or a new class of drugs. In lead optimization, it's also critical to know how well known binders or docking hits fulfil or violate the receptor's complementarity. One component of molecular modelling is molecular mechanics, which refers to the use of classical/Newtonian mechanics to describe the physical basis of the models. In most molecular models, atoms (the nucleus and electrons combined) are described as point charges with a mass. Spring-like interactions (representing chemical bonds) and Van der Waals forces describe the interactions between nearby atoms. The Lennard-Jones potential is often used to characterise Van der Waals forces. Coulomb's law is used to calculate electrostatic interactions. Atoms are given coordinates in Cartesian space or internal coordinates, and in dynamical simulations, they can also be given velocities. The atomic velocities are proportional to the system's temperature (a macroscopic quantity). A potential function is a mathematical expression that is related to the system's internal energy (U), which is equal to the sum of potential and kinetic energies (a thermodynamic quantity). Energy reduction techniques (e.g., steepest descent and conjugate gradient) are used to reduce potential energy, whereas molecular dynamics methods are used to predict the behaviour of a system with time propagation [120–130].

As previously stated, molecular docking's role in drug design has been divided into two paradigms: one focused on the structure-activity problem, which attempts to rationalise in the absence of detailed 3D structural information about the receptor, and the other focused on understanding the interaction seen in the receptor-ligand complex, which uses the known 3D structure of the therapeutic target to design novel drugs. A binding relationship between a small molecule ligand and an enzyme protein can cause the enzyme to be activated or inhibited. Ligand binding may cause agonism or antagonism if the protein is a receptor. The most common application of docking is in the field of medication design. The most medications are tiny organic compounds and docking may be applied as follows,

- *Hit identification*: Docking paired with a scoring algorithm can be used to swiftly screen vast databases of prospective medications using hit identification. To find compounds that are likely to bind to a protein target of interest *in silico* (virtual screening).

- *Lead optimization*: Docking can be used to anticipate whether and where a ligand binds to a protein in terms of relative orientation (also referred to as the binding mode or pose). This knowledge could be used to create more potent and selective analogues.

- *Bioremediation*: Protein ligand docking can be used to predict which contaminants enzymes can digest.

Molecular docking not only contributes to the design of potent compounds but also assist various steps in development of new drugs from laboratory to clinic. Few examples of contribution of molecular modeling are design of thimidylate synthetase inhibitors as anticancer agents, HIV protease inhibitors as antiviral agents, neutrophil elastase inhibitors as agents for emphysema, carbonic anhydrase inhibitors as antiglucoma agents and in discovery of novel sweeteners-taste receptor models [131–133]

In addition to the existing large number of docking programs, there are also many molecular mechanics programs applicable to these problems. Of course, there are some programs that are very widely used. Nevertheless it seems that the programs are not that easy to use and require some understanding of the underlying computational principles. Some of the software system are listed below [134–139].

Drug design targets	Molecules	Outcome (brand name of drugs and category)	Method employed	Research group
Thrombin inhibition	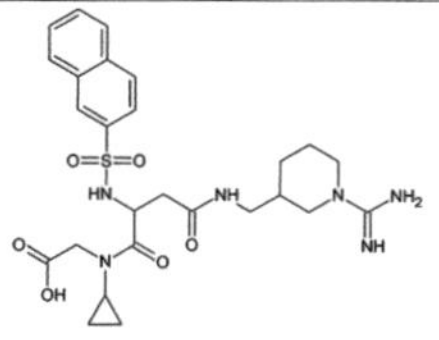 Napsagatran	Napsagatran: Direct thrombin inhibitor	Iterative cycles of modelling, synthesis and crystallography to optimise hydrophobic sites.	Hoffman-La Roache, Ltd.
Thrombin inhibition	[D-Phe-Pro-Arg-Pro-(Gly)4-Asn- Gly-Asp-Phe-Glu-Glu-Ile-Pro- Glu-Glu-Tyr-Leu] Bivalirudin	Bivalirudin: Thrombin inhibitor in cardiovascular events	Based on 3D model of thrombin, bifunctional peptide inhibitors were designed.	Biogen, Inc.
Neuramini-dase inhibition	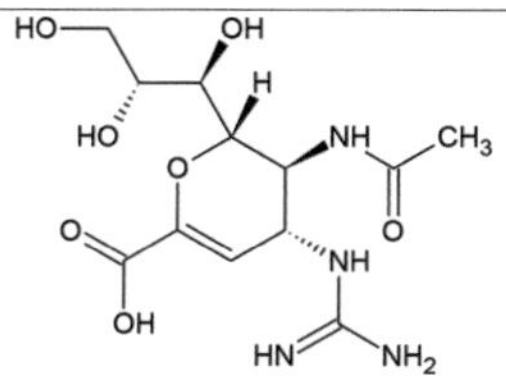 Desipramine	Desipramine: Treatment of irritable bowel syndrome, depression, vulvodynia, dysautonomia and effective against influenza A and B viruses	Use of primary amine probe from GRID for the neuraminidase binding site.	Monash University/G laxo Wellcome Lab.
Purine nucleoside phosphorrylase inhibition	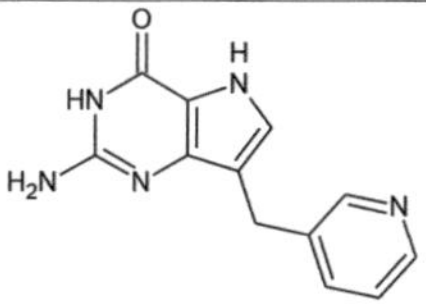 BCX-34 (Peldesine)	BCX-34: In HIV-infected patients and as an anticancer agent.	Modelling, synthesis and crystallography to screen synthetic candidates.	Biocryst pharmaceuti cals, Inc.
Thymidylate synthase inhibition	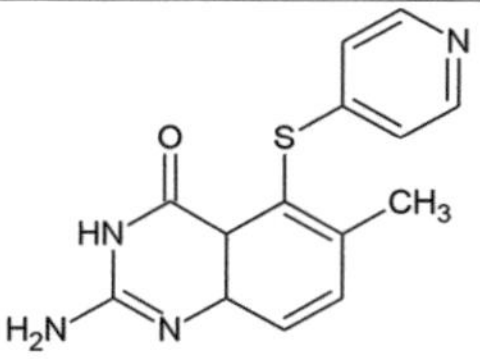 Thymitaq	Thymitaq, Nolatrexed: Treatment of leukaemia	Modelling, synthesis and crystallography to screen synthetic candidates. GRID program.	Agouron Pharmaceuti cals, Inc.
Carbonic anhydrase inhibition	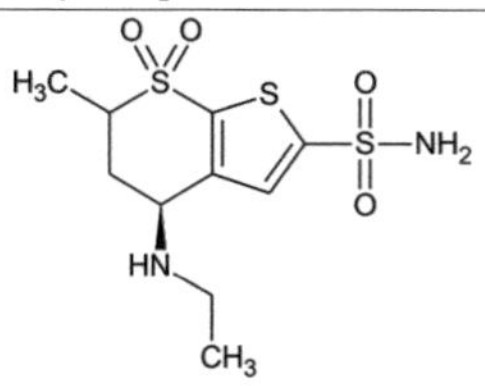 Dorzolamide	Dorzolamide: Inhibitor of carbonic anhydrase, inhibiting. Commonly used to treat glaucoma.	Multiple crystal structure determination combined with ab initio conformational analysis.	Merck Research Lab.
Human rhinovirus-14 inhibition	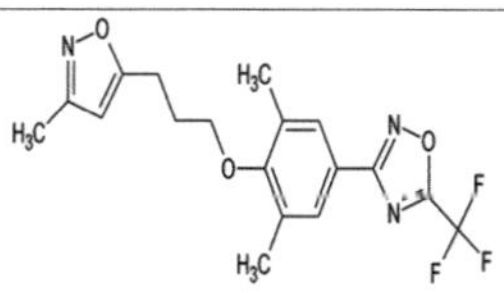 WIN 54954	WIN 54954: Made it past phase I clinical trial as a new broad-spectrum antipicornavirus drug, as a potential treatment of common cold.	Multiple crystal structure analysis and Volume map analysis	Sterling Winthrop Lab.

Drug design targets	Molecules	Outcome (brand name of drugs and category)	Method employed	Research group
Aldose reductase inhibition	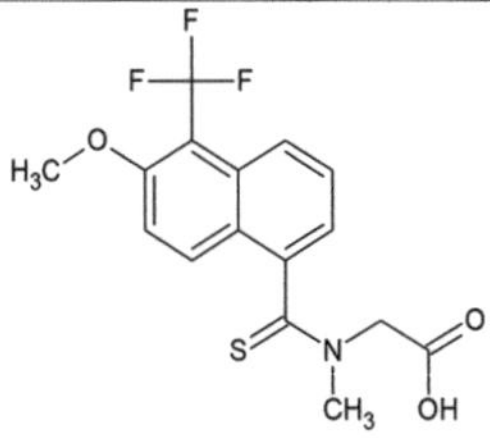 Tolrestat	Tolrestat: It was approved for marketed in several countries as antidiabetic agent. It was discontinued by Wyeth in 1997 because of the risk of severe liver toxicity and death.	Extended Huckel molecular orbital calculations, QSAR methodology	Ayerst Laboratories Research, Inc.

Table 2.
The successful application of computer assisted drug design approach to biological targets.

AutoDock: To generate a set of potential conformations, AutoDock use Monte Carlo simulated annealing and the LGA energy minimization is employed as a local search strategy and LGA is used as a global optimizer. The AMBER force field model is used in conjunction with free energy scoring functions and a wide set of protein-ligand complexes with known protein-ligand constants to analyse possible orientations. AutoDock's web pages are more informative than its competitors', and its free academic licence makes it a nice place to start if you're new to molecular docking software.

DOCK: DOCK is one of the most well-known and widely used ligand-protein docking tools. The initial version employed hard ligands; flexibility was later added by building the ligand in the binding pocket incrementally. DOCK, as previously stated, is a fragment-based technique that uses complimentary shape and chemistry methodologies to generate various ligand orientations. Three distinct scoring systems can be used to score these orientations; however, none of them include explicit hydrogen-bonding terms, solvation/desolvation words, or hydrophobicity parameters, limiting their usefulness. DOCK appears to handle polar binding sites well and is beneficial for quick docking, but it isn't the most precise programme available.

FlexX: FlexX is a fragment-based approach that uses hard proteins and flexible ligands. It creates conformers using the MIMUMBA torsion angle database. MIMUMBA is a database of intermolecular interaction patterns that uses interaction geometry to precisely define them. The Boehm function is used for scoring (with slight adjustments for docking). FlexX is used to emphasise the significance of scoring functions. Despite the fact that FlexX and DOCK are both fragment-based approaches, they give very distinct outputs. FlexX behaves in an entirely different way than DOCK, which works well with polar binding sites. It has a slightly lower hit rate than DOCK, but it produces superior Root Mean Square Distance estimates for compounds with accurately predicted binding modes. FlexE, a FlexX extension with flexible receptors, has been demonstrated to yield better outcomes with substantially shorter run times.

Gold: Because of its strong outcomes in independent tests, gold has gained a lot of new users in recent years. It has a good overall hit rate, although it struggles a little when dealing with hydrophobic binding pockets. To offer docking of a flexible ligand and a protein with flexible hydroxyl groups, Gold use a GA. Aside from that, the protein is considered stiff. When the binding pocket contains amino acids that create hydrogen bonds with the ligand, this makes it a favourable choice. Gold employs a scoring system based on favourable conformations discovered in the Cambridge Structural Database as well as empirical evidence on weak chemical interactions. The current focus of GOLD development is on enhancing the computational algorithm and introducing parallel processing capability.

3. Toxicity prediction and prediction adverse drug reaction

Any chemical's harmful or adverse effects are called as toxicity. Toxicity, such as carcinogenicity or genotoxicity, can be quantitative (e.g., lethal dose to 50% LD_{50} of tested individuals) or qualitative (e.g., toxic or nontoxic). In studies of toxicity the use of acute-exposure (single dose) or multiple-exposure (multiple dose) to determine detrimental effects of chemicals on humans, animals, plants, or the environment (multiple doses). Chemical toxicity is determine through several factors like the mode of exposure (oral, cutaneous or inhalation), dose, exposure frequency (single or multiple), exposure duration, qualities of chemical, biological properties (age, gender) and absorption, distribution, metabolism, excretion (ADME). Generally, animal models have been used for long time for toxicity testing. Nowadays advancements in high throughput screening, *in vitro* toxicity testing are easily achievable. Computational toxicology is one of the best toxicity assessment tool that establish, analyses, models, simulates, visualize or prediction of chemical toxicity. The simulation tools like algorithms, softwares, data, etc., which are projected *in vitro* toxicity experiments in order to avoid the animal models and cost effective toxicity testing which expands toxicity prediction and safety evaluation. Moreover, additional computational tools have the distinct benefits of being able to predict toxicity of substances even before they are created (**Figure 4**) [140].

Softwares (generating molecular descriptors):

- Simulation tools (systems biology and molecular dynamics)
- Modelling methods (toxicity prediction models)
- Statistical tools (generating prediction analysis)

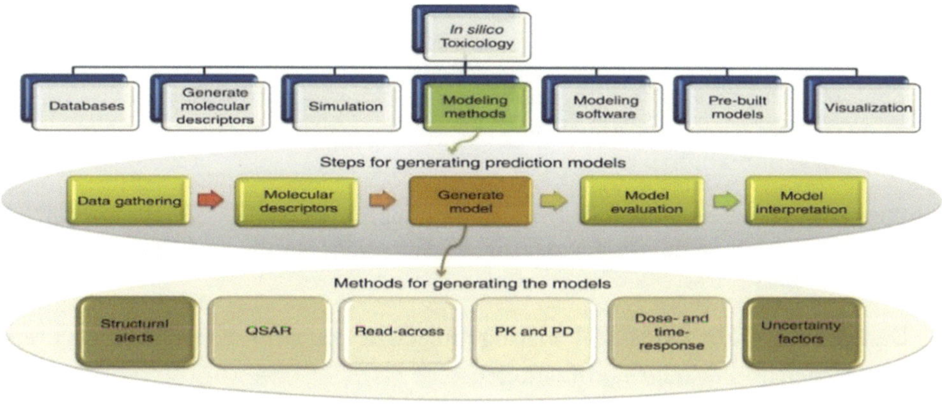

Figure 4.
In silico toxicology tools, steps to generate prediction models, and categories of prediction models [140].

- Expert system (include pre-built models in web serves or standalone application for predicting toxicity)

- Visualization tools

By and large, modeling approaches comprise five major steps while developing prediction models.

3.1 Why exploration of toxicity prediction is important?

Optimization of molecule is important during initial drug development for good efficacy as well as for pharmacokinetics (PKs) and toxicological properties prediction. Appropriate balance of target potency, selectivity, suitable ADME, and safe preclinical properties all together leads to the choice and clinical development of a potential new drug moiety. In clinical phase I trial the characteristic compound have to undergo years of preclinical testing and acquire only 8% chance of getting to the market. The failure of development of new drug cause by its toxicity. Therefore, executing toxicity analysis to be done in the early phase of the development process which gives significant potential to make value.

The major reasons that impede pharmaceutical companies to conduct earlier screening for toxicity like the big amount of compounds required for *in vivo* studies, the deficiency of *in vitro* assay predictions through high throughput along with inability of *in vitro* and animal models to proper prediction of toxicity in humans. The development of computational tools or *in silico* tools for prediction of toxicity are required to avoid above mentioned hurdles. These tools are structure based or using modeling techniques on human data, which provides approaches for removing the toxic effect in humans before the physical appearance of compound. The importance of computational tools arises from their applicability early in development stage. During the last few years, computational toxicology prediction system tremendously increased their forecasting ability but still unable to achieve the significant achievement because of deficit of big datasets contain toxicological effects like hepatotoxicity, teratogenicity, etc. The development of low throughput data with generations and coordinated efforts and set up on big historical background of experience and trained with small additional efforts may save a big investment and avoid use of animals (**Table 3**) [141].

- QSAR, expert systems, grouping and read-across techniques are used in structure activity modelling.

- Chemoinformatics: generating molecular descriptors for toxicity prediction using computational tools such as quantum chemical methods and molecular dynamics simulations;

- Databases and biological data that contain relationships between chemicals and toxicity endpoints, databases for storing data about chemicals, toxicity, and chemical properties;

- Data mining and analysis: calculating molecular descriptors, generating a prediction model, and evaluating the model;

Studies in laboratory animals have traditionally been used to determine the possible risks of chemicals, with modifications in clinical pathology and histology

In Silico **methods**	**Description**	**Software/databases**
Quantitative structure-activity relationship models	Use of molecular descriptors to predict chemical toxicity	OECD QSAR
		TopKat
		Derek Nexus
		VEGA
		METEOR
		vLife-QSARpro
Structural alerts and rule-based models	Chemical structures that indicate or associate to toxicity	OECD QSAR
		Toxtree
		OCES
		Derek Nexus
		HazardExpert
		Meteor
		CASE
		PASS
		cat-SAR
Read-across	Predicting unknown toxicity of a chemical using similar chemicals with known toxicity from the same chemical category	OECD QSAR
		Toxmatch
		ToxTree
		AMBIT
		AmbitDiscovery
		AIM
		DSSTox
		ChemIDplus
Dose–response and time–response models	Relation between doses (or time) and the incidence of a defined biological effect.	CEBS
		PubChem
		ToxRefDB
PK and pharmacodynamics (PD) models	PK models calculate concentration at a given time. PD models calculate effect at a given concentration	WinNonlin
		Kinetica
		ADAPT

Table 3.
In silico tools used for predicting toxicity endpoints of chemicals/drugs.

compared to untreated controls defining an adverse effect. In recent decades, there has been a greater degree of agreement in the definition of adversity in experimental animals caused by chemically produced effects, as well as in the assessment of human relevance. More recently, a paradigm change in toxicity testing has been proposed, largely as a result of animal welfare concerns, but also as a result of the development of new technologies. *In vitro* methods, toxicogenomic technologies, and computational tools are already available to provide mechanistic insight into the toxicological mode of action (MOA) of deleterious effects found in laboratory animals. Tox21c (toxicity testing in the twenty first century) is an idea that intends to forecast *in vivo* toxicity using a bottom-up strategy, starting with an understanding of MOA based on *in vitro* data and eventually predicting detrimental effects in humans [142].

Data sets and metrics used for drug side effect prediction:

- Important data sets for drug side effect prediction
- Metrics for drug side effect prediction
- Literature survey
  - Docking-based approaches
  - Network-based approaches
  - Machine learning-based approaches

Figure 5 depicts the categorization as well as the numerous approaches within each of the categories. The next sections discuss each of these categories and describe some of the most important efforts in the field of drug side effect prediction that have been done in each of these categories.

- *Docking-based approaches:* The preferred orientation of one molecule with another to form a stable compound is referred to as docking. Docking is one of the most used strategies for designing drugs based on structural data. The ability of targets to bind to one another is a critical property that impacts the efficiency of biochemical processes. When a medicine attaches to a certain protein, it can produce side effects. Drug side effect prediction using docking-based techniques

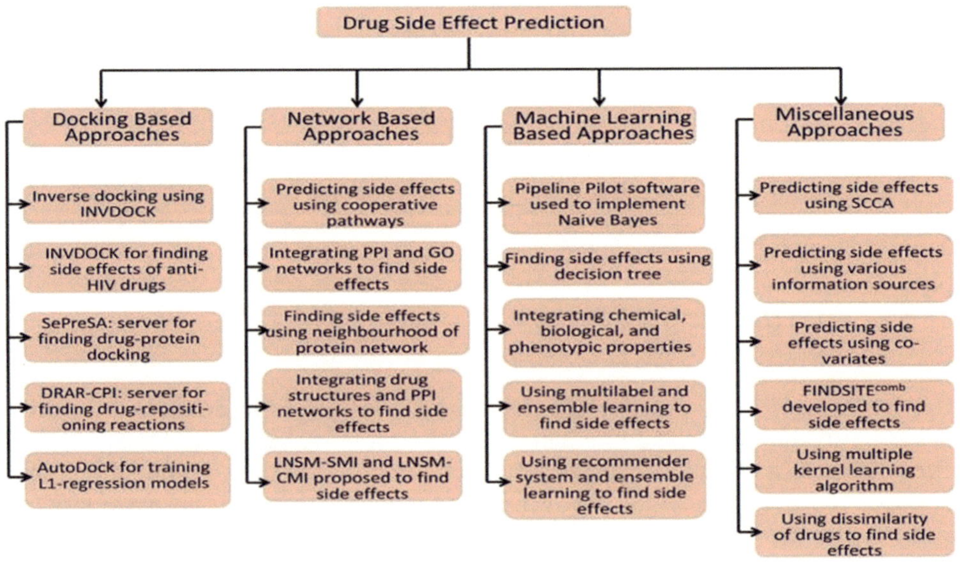

Figure 5.
Classification of drug side effect prediction approaches [143].

identifies possible drug binding sites. Many adverse effects are thought to be caused by an unexpected interaction of a medication molecule with a specific protein [144]. Side effects occur when a medication molecule is overregulated or communicates with a protein in an unexpected way. A molecular docking-based method for finding these target proteins has been presented INVDOCK. Various side effect–protein relationships were discovered during the method's evaluation. Various publications supporting the indicated side effect–protein relationships were discovered by searching the PubMed data collection.

- *Network-based approaches*: Drugs, targets, and side effects are viewed as nodes in a graph by networks. Edges are used to represent nodes. This graph-based visualization is used in network-based approaches to side effect prediction to identify pharmacological side effects. Side effects are induced by a variety of circumstances, including incorrect dose, binding to non-targets, and insufficient metabolization among others. To gain a better understanding of the factors that influence a disease, the actions of pharmaceuticals and their accompanying side effects, chemical substances, and associated targets are seen as a network.

- *Machine learning-based approaches*: Machine learning encompasses a variety of strategies and algorithms for gaining access to data and using it to learn about a certain area. Based on the training data, the various machine learning classifiers divide the observations into different classes. Machine learning-based approaches, on the other hand, use a variety of classifiers to solve the prediction problem. To improve prediction efficiency, the employment of SVM, naive Bayes, RF, and other methods has been recommended. In addition, as compared to other methods, machine learning-based methods take up less computing time. As a result, they can be used in post-market drug screening.

- *Miscellaneous approaches*: Miscellaneous approaches also provide valuable interaction prediction strategies. The SCCA-based method is also efficient in terms of computing time. Diverse scoring systems are used to quantify the chance of medicinal compounds interacting with their protein targets in various techniques to predict pharmacological side effects. The scoring approaches are effective in terms of computational complexity.

4. Polypharmacology and drug repositioning

Polypharmacology, a new paradigm in drug discovery that focuses on multi-target medicines (MTDs), has applications in drug repurposing, the process of finding new uses for already-approved pharmaceuticals, off-target toxicology prediction, and rational MTD design. In this situation, computational approaches have shown great promise in predicting polypharmacology and assisting with pharmaceutical repurposing [145].

The goal of polypharmacology is to identify a small ligands with off-target activities. Polypharmacology and chemogenomics have a high level of interaction. Chemogenomics is the study of the relationship between targets and their ligands in terms of structure and activity. The information about a target's ligands and its distance from other targets in biological space can be used to aid in the evaluation of new compounds for one or more novel targets. Both approaches can be employed in the early stages of development to screen out compounds and reduce the probability of failure due to significant adverse effects. When used on known medications, polypharmacological approaches can lead to a compound's repurposing for a new indication. Drug repurposing is suitable for marketed medications or development candidates that have failed in clinical trials due to lack of efficacy but have a strong safety profile and PK features [146]. Because prior clinical trial studies provide valuable data on drug PKs/PDs and toxicity profiles, repurposing previously approved pharmaceuticals saves time and money in drug development when compared to generating novel drugs from scratch. Sildenafil (Viagra®), a medicine that was originally created to treat hypertension but is now marketed to treat penile erection dysfunction, is a well-known example of drug repositioning [147].

Most pharmaceutical corporations and specialized service providers are increasing their medication repurposing activities in response to the present productivity problem and the need to minimize attrition rates in drug development. Because large pharmaceutical corporations, in particular, have a large pool of unsuccessful drug candidates, dedicated divisions have been formed and collaboration agreements have been negotiated. As a result of the endeavour, there has been a rise in the development and application of *in silico* approaches in this field. Due to computational constraints, *in silico* approaches for polypharmacology analysis and medication repurposing have primarily relied on 2D representations of small compounds. First, 3D approaches have already been outlined, but further research will allow for the discovery of target-target correlations that are not conceivable in the 2D world. This, together with recent breakthroughs in 3D tool computational throughput, suggests that these methods will be able to be used on the same scale as 2D tools in the near future [148]. Because of its potential applications and recent successes, polypharmacology has inspired a lot of interest in drug discovery [149]. Polypharmacology is exemplified by kinase inhibitors. Imatinib, for example, was developed to target the BCR-ABL protein and was licenced by the Food and Drug Administration to treat chronic myelogenous leukaemia [150].

High-throughput virtual screening (HTVS) is a simple tool for detecting hits in a single-target drug discovery project, but it is insufficient when several targets are investigated at the same time. In order to address polypharmacology, a multi-target approach must be developed. In order to identify the "magic shotgun" that can target numerous receptors at the same time, inverse docking techniques must be used. This enables the bioactivity and secondary effects of a potential new drug to be predicted, as well as the repositioning of existing treatments. Polypharmacology of known drugs and novel compounds is predicted *in silico* using structure-based and ligand-based approaches, as well as the rational design of MTDs.

In silico approaches have advanced as a valuable strategy in early drug development, and as additional target structures, structural bioactivity data, and therefore enhanced chemoinformatic tools become accessible, their influence will certainly grow. Because medications with a certain polypharmacologic profile will allow for better treatment of certain diseases, one of the most important computational challenges ahead is the application and development of algorithms for identifying suitable molecules (**Figure 6**).

Polypharmacology can be predicted using computational methods. Statistical data analysis and bioinformatics, ligand-based, and structure-based approaches can be used singly or in combination to take use of each approach's unique characteristics and strengths. The figure's lower half depicts three separate proteins (A–C) interacting with the same ligand, emphasising that the ligand's final pharmacological effect is the product of synergistic effects emerging from interactions with all targets.

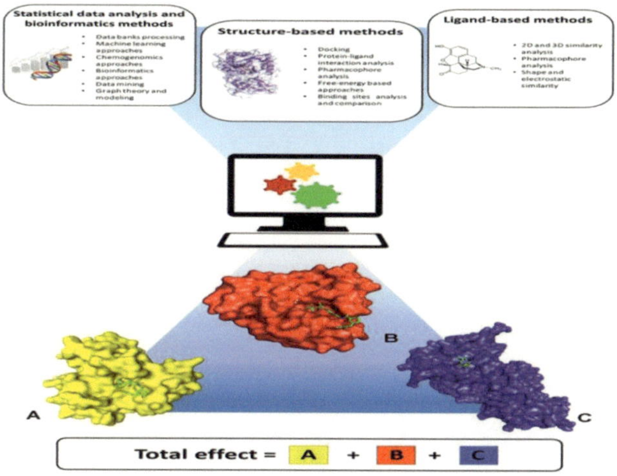

Figure 6.
Polypharmacology can be predicted using computational methods [148].

Structure-based approaches, ligand-based methods, and systems biology methods are the three categories of methodologies that can be used to anticipate unknown targets for small compounds.

- *Structure-based methods*: Inverse docking, binding site similarities, inverse pharmacophore modelling, molecular dynamics simulations, and fragment-based multi-target drug design are examples of structure-based techniques. Currently, the Protein Data Bank (PDB) has substantially includes 3D protein structures that refined by protein crystallography, nuclear magnetic resonance spectroscopy, and electron microscopy. Due to the availability of such structural data, inverse docking algorithms have been developed, with the primary goal of docking a small molecule into binding sites of many targets for hit identification. INVDOCK, TarFisDock, and idTarget are some of the modified scoring functions that have been developed specifically for target ranking in recent years. Binding site similarity-based search, in addition to inverse docking, is commonly employed for target prediction. It's based on the idea that structurally comparable proteins have similar chemical functions, thus they'll probably bind to structurally similar substances. Combining the GRID Molecular Interaction Fields with pharmacophoric characteristics, the Fingerprints for Ligands and Proteins (FLAP) algorithm was recently developed. Drug repurposing and hit identification can both benefit from binding site similarity technologies. It can also be employed in the lead optimization process by comparing binding locations. Advanced pharmacophore approaches have recently been developed to connect structure-based pharmacophore models of targets with small molecule pharmacophoric features to small molecule pharmacophoric features. Fragments are smaller, simpler chemical entities than drug/lead-like compounds, and they have a higher promiscuous nature. Fragment-based techniques boost the likelihood of obtaining hits and aid in the discovery of novel compounds because a small number of pieces can cover a large chemical search area. As a result, they can be utilised for hit detection, lead generation, and lead optimization.

- *Ligand-based methods*: The characteristics and activities of compounds are used to anticipate unknown targets utilising ligand-based techniques. This is based on the notion that structurally similar molecules attach to similar targets. The similarity ensemble approach (SEA) is a similarity-based method for determining the likelihood of a molecule binding to a target based on topological similarities between the ligands. Recently smooth surface triangulator (SMART) algorithm, pair-wise kernel method (PKM), Gaussian interaction profile, Laplacian regularized least squares (LapRLS), kernel regression, kernelized Bayesian matrix factorization with twin kernels (KBMF2K), and bipartite local method have been developed.

- *Systems biology methods*: With the development of high-throughput techniques yielding massive amounts of data in domains like genomics and proteomics, understanding diseases, especially complex ones, has never been more detailed. The term "Network Pharmacology" was coined to propose that combining chemogenomics data with network biology might aid in the development of new ways to target disease-causing networks rather than specific genes or targets. The database, which contains over millions of drug-induced gene expression patterns, can be utilised to find new polypharmacology medicines.

The concept that comparable drugs bind to similar targets still underpins the majority of polypharmacology research. The development of precise and robust scoring algorithms that can rank targets rather than tiny molecules is a big challenge. Novel approaches to rational design of multi-targeting small molecules are now being investigated. Apart from traditional structure- and ligand-based approaches, there has been an upsurge in interest in system biology and bioinformatics-based methodologies, as well as community-wide activities. These approaches have been demonstrated to not only anticipate new small molecule targets, but also to aid in the understanding of disease dynamics and the molecular interaction pathways that lie beneath. Polypharmacology, which can predict both on-target and off-target therapeutic effects, could help in illness targeting. As a result, the rational polypharmacological drug design (PDD) holds a lot of promise and possibility for drug discovery in the future. However, in order to reach such ambitious aims and, eventually, translate information into successful patient therapy, we must overcome a number of flaws and roadblocks [151].

The field of computational polypharmacology has progressed to the point where concrete hypotheses may be formulated using prediction results to guide wet-lab research. The field of computational polypharmacology has advanced to the point where concrete hypotheses may be established and used to guide wet lab research utilizing prediction results. Furthermore, the majority of contemporary approaches are implemented as web servers or standalone applications. As community efforts become more essential, it will be necessary to create portable programming libraries that community developers can use to alter existing toolkits or create new ones. More cell-free, cell-based, and animal models are needed in experimental assays to examine the impact of drugs on various targets or functions at the same time.

5. Opportunities and challenges

There are six components to the CADD challenges. Chemical and biological space are the two major categories. The term "chemical space" refers to the large number

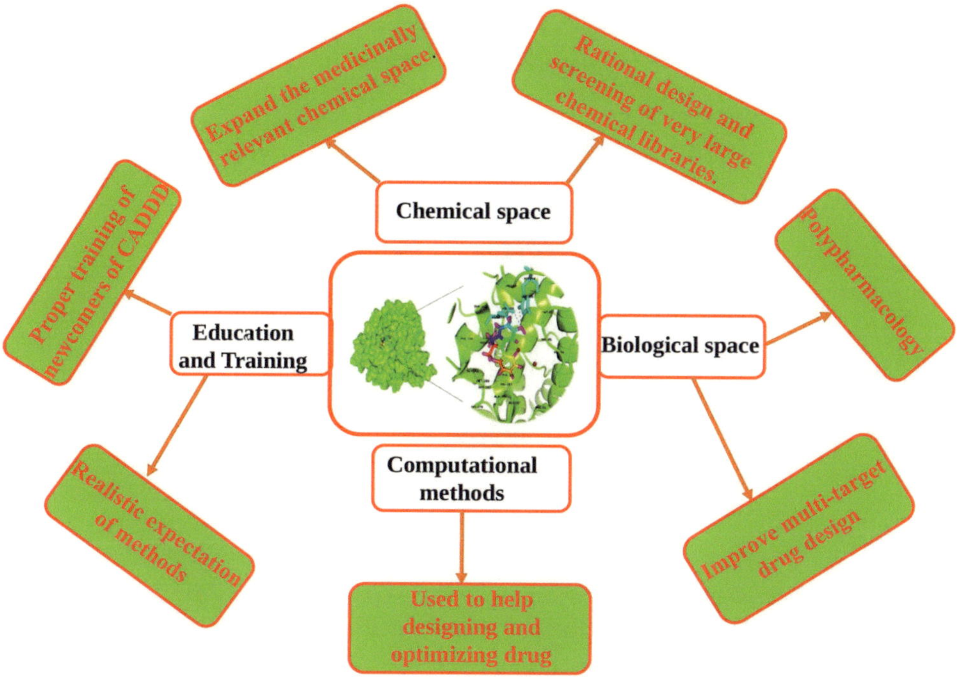

Figure 7.
In silico methods showing outstanding challenges during drug discovery and design.

of possibilities for discovering hit substances. Third is methodologies challenges, in which for designing and optimizing drug candidate's computational methods could be used. Last one is the proper training of newcomers like investigators of CADD for multidisciplinary work (**Figure 7**) [152–155].

The topic of drug repurposing is gaining impetus toward novel therapeutic molecule development, aided by an ever-increasing number of innovative computational techniques and enormous sequencing databases. Antibiotic resistance among key clinical pathogens is a grim prospect, as per infection-related death rate continues to rise despite a slowing rate of new antibiotic discovery.

6. Applications and limitations

CADD is useful in the treatment of neurodegenerative disorders particularly targeting Amyloid-β in case of Alzheimer's disease. For nearly two decades, in pharmaceutical research docking calculations have been used. Virtual screening using protein templates differs from virtual screening approaches based on molecular similarity and ligands beneficial for de novo identification of active complex. Three important factors in CADD pays close attention include: (1) As per target structure, screening a large number of molecules, which can then be assessed using both experimental and computational techniques; (2) as per affinity, criteria on toxicity and PK study, guiding the optimization of lead compounds and (3) based on the structure, supporting in the design of novel compounds to recover functions of drug. For modelling of drug the CADD approach is extremely helpful. Computed chemistry and bioinformatics, as well as combinatorial chemistry, are used to handle the many issues connected

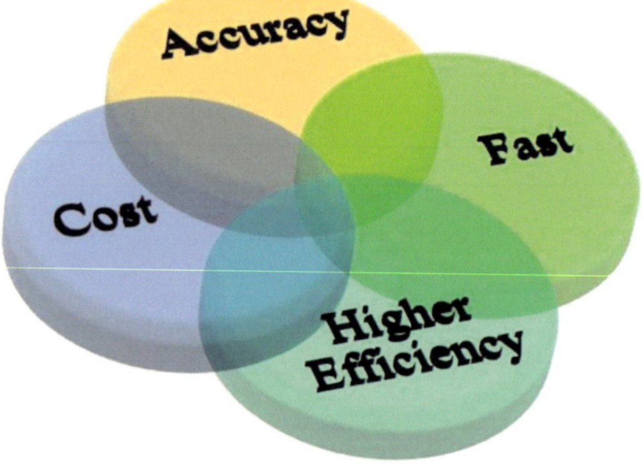

Figure 8.
Advantages of CADD.

with the drug discovery pipeline in less time and expense. As per **Figure 8**, general advantages of CADD are found to be cost effective, with higher efficiency, speed and accuracy in results [156–159].

FDA approved drugs like human immunodeficiency virus (HIV)-1-inhibiting drugs identified by SBDD available on the market. Other example is thymidylate synthase inhibitor, raltitrexed, by protein modelling, inhibitor of HIV protease, amprenavir is discovered. Computer assisted techniques are hypothetical and results must be confirmed in real-world systems, and pharmacological activities discovered through CADD in lead compounds have failed. Most of the methods of CADD methods like QSAR, molecular dynamics, molecular docking, etc. have their specific

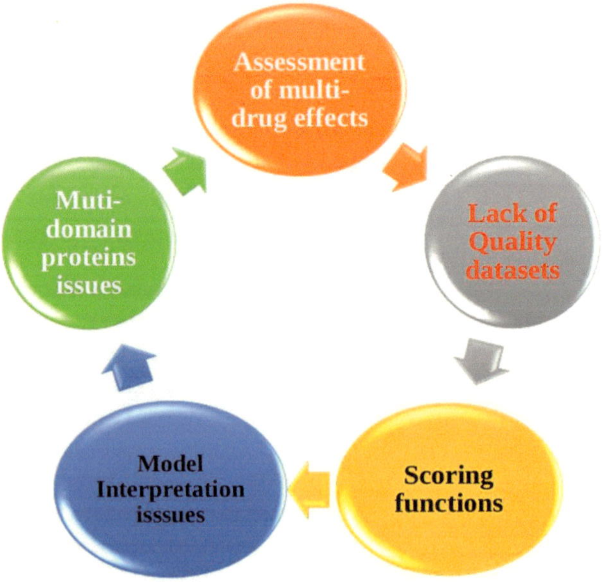

Figure 9.
Limitations of CADD.

restrictions. Limitations are found to be multi-domain protein issues that means protein flexibility which is the most problematic challenge, assessment of multi-drug effects, in some cases lack of quality datasets observed (**Figure 9**).

One failure example of SBDD is RPX00023 which was reported as an antidepressant activity as an agonist of the 5-HT1A receptor. However, it was found to be an inhibitors of 5-HT1A receptor [160–164].

Conflict of interest

We confirm that there is no conflict of interest.

Author details

Kishor Danao[1*], Deweshri Nandurkar[1], Vijayshri Rokde[1], Ruchi Shivhare[1] and Ujwala Mahajan[2]

1 Department of Pharmaceutical Chemistry, Dadasaheb Balpande College of Pharmacy, Nagpur, Maharashtra, India

2 Department of Quality Assurance, Dadasaheb Balpande College of Pharmacy, Nagpur, Maharashtra, India

*Address all correspondence to: kerzarepritee@gmail.com

References

[1] Houston JG, Banks MN. In: Abraham DJ, editor. Burger's Medicinal Chemistry and Drug Discovery. 6th ed. Hoboke, New Jersey: Wiley-Interscience; 2003. p. 38

[2] Camille G, Wermuth CG. The Practice of Medicinal Chemistry. London: Academic Press; 1996. p. 4

[3] Martin YC, Kuffer E, Austel A. Modern Drug Research, Paths to Better and Safer Drugs. New York: Marcel Dekker Inc; 1989. pp. 243-273

[4] Trickle IJ, Sibanda BL, Pearl CH, Hemming AM, Blundell TL. X-Ray Crystallography and Drug Action. Oxford: Clarendon Press; 1984. pp. 427-440

[5] Greer J, Erickson JW, Baldwin JJ, Varney MD. Application of the three-dimensional structures of protein target molecules in structure-based drug design. Journal of Medicinal Chemistry. 1994;**37**(8):1035-1054

[6] Tollenaere JP. In: Gund P, editor. Guidebook on Molecular Modeling in Drug Design. New York: Academic Press; 1996. p. 352

[7] Ariens EJ. Molecular Pharmacology. New York: Academic Press; 1964. p. 176

[8] Glenn S. In: Osol A, editor. Remington's Pharmaceutical Sciences. 16th ed. Easton, Pennsylvania: Mack Publishing Company; 1980. p. 8

[9] Webb ML. In: Gennaro AR, editor. Remington: The Science and Practice of Pharmacy. Vol. I. 20th ed. Philadelphia: Lippincott Williams and Wilkins; 2000. p. 81

[10] Newall C. In: Roberts S, Price B, editors. Medicinal Chemistry - The role of Organic Chemistry in Drug Research. 1st ed. London: Academic Press; 1985. p. 209

[11] Sternbach LH, Kaiser S. Antispasmodic. II. Esters of basic bicyclic alcohols. Journal of the American Chemical Society. 1952;**74**:2219-2221

[12] Treves GR, Testa FC. Basic esters and quaternary derivatives of β-hydroxy acids as antispasmodics. Journal of the American Chemical Society. 1952;**74**:46-48

[13] Tilford CH. Aminoesters of substituted alicyclic carboxylic acids. Journal of the American Chemical Society. 1947;**69**:2902-2906

[14] Karczmar AG. Ganglionic Blocking and Stimulating Agents. International Encyclopedia of Pharmacology and Therapeutics. Vol. I. Oxford: Pergamon Press; 1966. p. 342

[15] Hou JP, Poole JW. β-Lactam antibiotics: Their physicochemical properties and biological activities in relation to structure. Journal of Pharmaceutical Sciences. 1971;**60**:503-532

[16] Mayersohn M, Endrenyi L. Relative bioavailability of commercial ampicillin formulations in man. Canadian Medical Association Journal. 1973;**109**:989-993

[17] Hill SA, Jones KH, Seager H, Taskis CB. Dissolution and bioavailability of the anhydrate and trihydrate forms of ampicillin. The Journal of Pharmacy and Pharmacology. 1975;**27**:594-598

[18] Fong I, Engelking ER, Kirbi WM. Relative inactivation by *Staphylococcus aureus* of eight cephalosporin

antibiotics. Antimicrobial Agents and Chemotherapy. 1976;**9**:939-944

[19] Yamana T, Tsuji A. Comparative stability of cephalosporins in aqueous solution: Kinetics and mechanisms of degradation. Journal of Pharmaceutical Sciences. 1976;**65**:1563-1574

[20] Neu HC, Aswapokee N, Fu KP, Aswapokee P. Antibacterial activity of a new 1-oxa cephalosporin compared with that of other beta-lactam compounds. Antimicrobial Agents and Chemotherapy. 1979;**16**:141-149

[21] Domagk GJ. Ein Beitrag zur Chemotherapie der bakteriellen Infektionen. Deutsche Medizinische Wochenschrift. 1935;**61**:250-253

[22] Anand N. In: Wolff ME, editor. Burger's Medicinal Chemistry and Discovery. 5th ed. Vol. Vol. II. New York: Wiley-Interscience; 1996. p. 255

[23] Macdonald L, kazanijan, P. Opportunistic infections in patients with AIDS - treatment and prophylaxis. Formulary. 1996;**31**:470

[24] Jawetz E. In: Katzung BG, editor. Basic and Clinical Pharmacology. 6th ed. Norwalk, CT: Appleton and Lange; 1995. p. 478

[25] Shepard CC. Leprosy today. The New England Journal of Medicine. 1982;**307**:1640-1641

[26] Miner NA, McDowell JW, Willcockson GW, Bruckner NI, Stark RL, Whitmore EJ. Antimicrobial and other properties of a new stabilized alkaline glutaraldehyde disinfectant/sterilizer. American Journal of Hospital Pharmacy. 1977;**34**:376-382

[27] Domagala JM. Structure-activity and structure-side-effect relationships for the quinolone antibacterials. Antimicrobial Agents and Chemotherapy. 1994;**33**: 685-706

[28] Heifets LB, Flory MA, Lindholm-Levy P. Does pyrazinoic acid as an active moiety of pyrazinamide have specific activity against *Mycobacterium tuberculosis*? Antimicrobial Agents and Chemotherapy. 1989;**33**:1252-1254

[29] Werli W. Rifampin: Mechanisms of action and resistance. Reviews of Infectious Diseases. 1983;**55**:407-411

[30] Hartmann GR. Molecular mechanism of action of the antibiotic rifampicin. Angewandte Chemie (International Ed. in English). 1985;**24**:1009-1014

[31] Zhang Y, Heym B, Allen B, Young D, Cole S. The catalase-peroxidase gene and isoniazid resistance of *Mycobacterium tuberculosis*. Nature. 1992;**358**:591-593

[32] Scherrer RA. In: Scherrer RA, Whitehouse MW, editors. Anti-Inflammatory Agents. New York: Academic Press; 1974. p. 132

[33] Dornan J, Reynolds W. Comparison of ibuprofen and acetylsalicylic acid in the treatment of rheumatoid arthritis. Canadian Medical Association Journal. 1974;**110**:1370-1372

[34] Brogden RN, Heel RC, Speight TM, Avery GS. Fenoprofen: A review of its pharmacological properties and therapeutic efficacy in rheumatic disease. Drugs. 1977;**13**:241-265

[35] Chernish SM, Rosenak BD, Brunelie RL, Crabtree R. Comparison of gastrointestinal effects of aspirin and fenoprofen. Arthritis and Rheumatism. 1979;**22**:376-383

[36] Winters WD, Ferrar AT, Guzman FC, Alcaraz M. The cataleptic

state induced by ketamine: A review of the neuropharmacology of anesthesia. Neuropharmacology. 1972;**11**:303-315

[37] Greenblatt DJ, Shader RI. Benzodiazepine in Clinical Practice. New York: Raven Press; 1974. p. 17

[38] Greenblatt DJ, Shader RI, Abernethy DR. Drug therapy: Current status of benzodiazepines. Part One. New England Journal of Medicine. 1983;**309**:354-358

[39] Gastaut H, Broughton R. Anticonvulsant drugs. In: Radouco-Thomas C, editor. International Encyclopedia of Pharmacology and Therapeutics. Vol. I. New York: Pergamon Press; 1973. p. 3

[40] Spinks A, Waring WS. In: Ellis GP, West GB, editors. Progress in Medicinal Chemistry. Vol. III. Washington, DC: Butterworth; 1963. p. 345

[41] Hanka LJ, Evans JS, Mason DJ, Dietz A. Microbiological production of 5-azacytidine. I. Production and biological activity. Antimicrobial Agents and Chemotherapy. 1966;**6**:619-624

[42] Schaeffer HJ, Schwender CF. Enzyme inhibitors. 26. Bridging hydrophobic and hydrophilic regions on adenosine deaminase with some 9-(2-hydroxy-3-alkyl) adenines. Journal of Medicinal Chemistry. 1974;**17**:6-8

[43] Eckle E, Stezowski JJ. The crystal and molecular structure of 7-con-O-methylnogarol. Tetrahedron Letters. 1980;**21**:507-510

[44] Fujiwara K, Hiromi S, Masahiro H. Enyne[3]cumulene. Synthesis and mode of aromatization. The Journal of Organic Chemistry. 1991;**56**:1688-1689

[45] Harrison RC, McAuliffe CA. An efficient route for the preparation of highly soluble platinum (II) antitumour agents. Inorganica Chimica Acta. 1980;**46**:L15-L16

[46] Levitzki A, Gazit A. Tyrosine kinase inhibition: An approach to drug development. Science. 1995;**267**:1782-1788

[47] Moller JV, Sheikh MI. Renal organic anion transport system: Pharmacological, physiological and biochemical aspects. Pharmacological Reviews. 1983;**34**:315-356

[48] Mann T, Keilin K. Sulphanilamide as a specific inhibitor of carbonic anhydrase. Nature. 1940;**146**:164-165

[49] Leaf A, Cotran RS. In: Leaf A, Cortan RS, editors. Renal Pathophysiology. 2nd ed. New York: Oxford University Press; 1980. p. 145

[50] Shinkawa T, Fumiaki Y, Notsu T, Nakakuki M, Nishijima K, Yoshitomi K, et al. Loop and distal actions of a novel diuretic, M17055. European Journal of Pharmacology. 1993;**238**:317-325

[51] Cragoe EJ. In: Cragoe EJ, editor. Chemistry, Pharmacology and Medicine. New York: John Wiley and Sons; 1983. p. 303

[52] Roberts LS, Schmidt GD. Foundations of Parasitology. USA: William C Brown Pub; 1995. p. 324

[53] Hardman JG, Limbiad LE. The Pharmacological Basis of Therapeutics. 9th ed. New York: Macmillan; 1996. p. 576

[54] Foye WO. In: Foye WO, Lemke TL, Williams DA, editors. Principles of Medicinal Chemistry. 4th ed. Philadelphia: Lea and Febiger; 1995. p. 348

[55] Banks BJ. Antiparasitic agents. In: Bailey DM, editor. Annual Reports in Medicinal Chemistry. Vol. 19. New York: Academic Press; 1984. p. 198

[56] Cox FEG. Which way for malaria? Nature. 1988;**332**:486-487

[57] Walsh C. Antibiotics: Actions, Origins, Resistance. 1st ed. New York: ASM Press; 1956. pp. 223-324

[58] Mechlinski W, Schaffner CP, Ganis P, Avitabile G. Structure and absolute configuration of the polyene macrolide antibiotic amphotericin B. Tetrahedron Letters. 1970;**11**:3873-3876

[59] Pandey RC, Rinehart K. Carbon-13 nuclear magnetic resonance evidence for cyclic hemiketals in the polyene antibiotics amphotericin B, nystatin A1, tetrin A, tetrin B, lucensomycin and pimaricin 1,2. The Journal of Antibiotics. 1976;**29**:1035-1342

[60] Mitscher LA, Sharma PM, Chu DT, Shen LL, Pernet AG. Chiral DNA gyrase inhibitors 2. Asymmetric synthesis and biological activity of the enantiomers of 9-fluoro-3-methyl-10-(4-methyl-1-piperazinyl)-7-oxo-2,3-dihydro-7h-pyrido[1,2,3-de]-1,4-benzoxazine-6-carboxylic acid (ofloxacin). Journal of Medicinal Chemistry. 1987;**30**:2283-2286

[61] Garrison JC. In: Gilman AG, Rall TW, Nies AS, Taylor P, editors. Goodman and Gilman's The Pharmacological Basis of Therapeutics. 8th ed. New York: Pergamon Press; 1990. p. 398

[62] Mann KV, Crowe JP, Tietze KJ. Non sedating histamine H1-receptor antagonists. Clinical Pharmacy. 1989;**8**:331-344

[63] Barouh V, Dall H, Patel D, Hite G. Stereochemical aspects of antihistamine action. 4. Absolute configuration of carbinoxamine antipodes. Journal of Medicinal Chemistry. 1971;**14**:834-836

[64] Leurs R, Timmerman H. Progress in Drug Research. Vol. 39. Boston: Virkhauser Verlag; 1992. p. 127

[65] Saxena AK. Saxena M. In: Jucker E, editor. Progress in Drug Research. Vol. 39. Boston: Birkhauser Verlag; 1992. p. 35

[66] Wermuth CG. Drug Design-Fact or Fantasy. 1st ed. New York: Academic Press; 1984. p. 47

[67] Gerhard K, Abrahum UJ. Comparative molecular similarity index analysis (CoMSIA) to study hydrogen bonding properties and to store combinatorial libraries. Computer Aided Molecular Design. 1999;**13**:1-10

[68] Venger BH, Hanch C, Hathwan GJ, Amerein YV. Ames-test of 1-(X-phenyl)-3,3-dialkyl triazines. A quantitative structure activity study. Journal of Medicinal Chemistry. 1979;**22**:473-476

[69] Carter RC, Grassy G, Kubinyl H, Martin YC, Willett P. Chapter 37. Glossary of terms used in computational drug design (IUPAC Recommendations 1997). Annual Reports in Medicinal Chemistry. 1998;**33**:397-409

[70] Propst CL, Perun TJ. In: Marcel D, Perun TJ, Propst CK, editors. Computer Aided Drug Design Methods and Application. New York: Marcel Dekker Inc; 1989. p. 12

[71] Leow GH, Villar HO, Alkorta I. Strategies for indirect computer-aided drug design. Pharmaceutical Research. 1993;**10**:475-486

[72] Workman P. How much gets there and what does it do?: The need for better

pharmacokinetic and pharmacodynamic endpoints in contemporary drug discovery and development. Current Pharmaceutical Design. 2003;**9**:891-902

[73] Stahura FL, Bajorath J. virtual screening methods that complement HTS. Combinatorial Chemistry & High Throughput Screening. 2004;7:259-269

[74] Guner O, Clement O, Kurogi Y. Pharmacophore modeling and three dimensional database searching for drug design using catalyst: Recent advances. Current Medicinal Chemistry. 2004;**11**:2991-3005

[75] Leo AJ, Hansch C. Role of hydrophobic effects in mechanistic QSAR. Perspectives in Drug Discovery and Design. 1999;**17**:1-25

[76] Bolis G, Dipace L, Fabrocini F. A machine learning approach to computer aided molecular design. Journal of Computer-Aided Molecular Design. 1991;**5**:617-628

[77] Zhang S, Du-Cuny L. Development and evaluation of a new statistical model for structure-based high-throughput virtual screening. International Journal of Bioinformatics Research and Applications. 2009;**5**:269-279

[78] Beusen DD, Marshall GR. In: Guner OF, editor. Pharmacophore Perception, Development, and Use in Drug Design. La Jolla, CA: International University Line; 2000. pp. 23-45

[79] Van Drie JH. "Shrink-Wrap" surfaces: A new method for incorporating shape into pharmacophoric 3D database searching. Journal of Chemical Information and Computer Sciences. 1997;**37**:38-42

[80] Patel Y, Gillet VJ, Bravi G, Leach AR. A comparison of the pharmacophore identification programs: Catalyst, DISCO and GASP. Journal of Computer-Aided Molecular Design. 2002;**16**:653-681

[81] Cho AE, Guallar V, Berne B, Friesner RA. Importance of accurate charges in molecular docking: Quantum mechanical/molecular mechanical (QM/MM) approach. Journal of Computational Chemistry. 2005;**26**:915-931

[82] Brint AT, Willett P. Algorithms for the identification of three-dimensional maximal common substructures. Journal of Chemical Information and Computer Sciences. 1987;**27**:152-158

[83] Fischer D, Norel R, Wolfson H, Nussinov R. Surface motifs by a computer vision technique: Searches, detection, and implications for protein-ligand recognition. Proteins. 1993;**16**(3):278-292

[84] Norel R, Fischer D, Wolfson HJ, Nussinov R. Molecular surface recognition by a computer vision-based technique. Protein Engineering. 1994;**7**(1):39-46

[85] Miller MD, Kearsley SK, Underwood DJ, Sheridan RP. FLOG: A system to select 'quasi-flexible' ligands complementary to a receptor of known three-dimensional structure. Journal of Computer-Aided Molecular Design. 1994;**8**(2):153-174

[86] Diller DJ, Merz KM Jr. High throughput docking for library design and library prioritization. Proteins. 2001;**43**(2):113-124

[87] Burkhard P, Taylor P, Walkinshaw MD. An example of a protein ligand found by database mining: Description of the docking method and its verification by a 2.3 A X-ray structure of a thrombin-ligand complex. Journal of Molecular Biology. 1998;**277**(2):449-466

[88] DesJarlais RL, Sheridan RP, Dixon JS, Kuntz ID, Venkataraghavan R. Docking flexible ligands to macromolecular receptors by molecular shape. Journal of Medicinal Chemistry. 1986;**29**(11):2149-2153

[89] Kuntz ID, Leach AR. Conformational analysis of flexible ligands in macromolecular receptor sites. Journal of Computational Chemistry. 1992;**13**:730-748

[90] Ewing TJ, Makino S, Skillman AG, Kuntz ID. DOCK 4.0: Search strategies for automated molecular docking of flexible molecule databases. Journal of Computer-Aided Molecular Design. 2001;**15**(5):411

[91] Welch W, Ruppert J, Jain AN. Hammerhead: Fast, fully automated docking of flexible ligands to protein binding sites. Chemistry & Biology. 1996;**3**(6):449-462

[92] Kollman PA. Free energy calculations: Applications to chemical and biochemical phenomena. Chemical Reviews. 1993;**93**:2395-2417

[93] Aqvist J, Luzhkov VB, Brandsdal BO. Ligand binding affinities from MD simulations. Accounts of Chemical Research. 2002;**35**(6):358-365

[94] Carlson HA, Jorgensen WL. An extended linear response method for determining free energies of hydration. The Journal of Physical Chemistry. 1995;**99**:10667-10673

[95] Shoichet BK, Stroud RM, Santi DV, Kuntz ID, Perry KM. Structure-based discovery of inhibitors of thymidylate synthase. Science. 1993;**259**(5100):1445-1450

[96] Michel J, Verdonk ML, Essex JW. Protein-ligand binding affinity predictions by implicit solvent simulations: A tool for lead optimization? Journal of Medicinal Chemistry. 2006;**49**(25):7427-7439

[97] Briggs JM, Marrone TJ, McCammon JA. Computational science new horizons and relevance to pharmaceutical design. Trends in Cardiovascular Medicine. 1996;**6**:198-206

[98] Gehlhaar DK, Verkhivker GM, Rejto PA, Sherman CJ, Fogel DB, Fogel LJ, et al. Molecular recognition of the inhibitor AG-1343 by HIV-1 protease: Conformationally flexible docking by evolutionary programming. Chemistry & Biology. 1995;**2**(5):317-324

[99] Verkhivker GM, Bouzida D, Gehlhaar DK, Rejto PA, Arthurs S, Colson AB, et al. Deciphering common failures in molecular docking of ligandprotein complexes. Journal of Computer-Aided Molecular Design. 2000;**14**(8):731-751

[100] Jain AN. Scoring noncovalent protein-ligand interactions: A continuous differentiable function tuned to compute binding affinities. Journal of Computer-Aided Molecular Design. 1996;**10**(5):427-440

[101] Head RD, Smythe ML, Oprea TI, Waller CL, Green SM, Marshall GR. VALIDATE: A new method for the receptor-based prediction of binding affinities of novel ligands. Journal of the American Chemical Society. 1996;**118**:3959-3969

[102] Gehlhaar DK, Moerder KE, Zichi D, Sherman CJ, Ogden RC, Freer ST. De novo design of enzyme inhibitors by Monte Carlo ligand generation. Journal of Medicinal Chemistry. 1995;**38**(3):466-472

[103] Eldridge MD, Murray CW, Auton TR, Paolini GV, Mee RP. Empirical

scoring functions: I. The development of a fast empirical scoring function to estimate the binding affinity of ligands in receptor complexes. Journal of Computer-Aided Molecular Design. 1997;**11**(5):425-445

[104] Muegge I, Martin YC. A general and fast scoring function for protein-ligand interactions: A simplified potential approach. Journal of Medicinal Chemistry. 1999;**42**(5):791-804

[105] Still WC, Tempczyk A, Hawley RC, Hendrickson T. Semianalytical treatment of solvation for molecular mechanics and dynamics. Journal of the American Chemical Society. 1990;**112**(16):6127-6129

[106] Guimaraes CR, Mathiowetz AM. Addressing limitations with the MM-GB/SA scoring procedure using the WaterMap method and free energy perturbation calculations. Journal of Chemical Information and Modeling. 2010;**50**(4):547-559

[107] Singh N, Warshel A. Absolute binding free energy calculations: On the accuracy of computational scoring of protein-ligand interactions. Proteins. 2010;**78**(7):1705-1723

[108] Gabb HA, Jackson RM, Sternberg MJ. Modelling protein docking using shape complementarity, electrostatics and biochemical information. Journal of Molecular Biology. 1997;**272**(1):106-120

[109] Bron C, Kerbosch J. Algorithm 457: Finding all cliques of an undirected graph. Communications of the ACM. 1973;**16**(9):575-576

[110] Meng EC, Shoichet BK, Kuntz ID. Automated docking with grid-based energy evaluation. Journal of Computational Chemistry. 1992;**13**:505-524

[111] Meng XY, Zheng QC, Zhang HX. A comparative analysis of binding sites between mouse CYP2C38 and CYP2C39 based on homology modeling, molecular dynamics simulation and docking studies. Biochimica et Biophysica Acta. 2009;**1794**(7):1066-1072

[112] Boehm HJ, Boehringer M, Bur D, Gmuender H, Huber W, Klaus W, et al. Novel inhibitors of DNA gyrase: 3D structure based biased needle screening, hit validation by biophysical methods, and 3D guided optimization. A promising alternative to random screening. Journal of Medicinal Chemistry. 2000;**43**(14):2664-2674

[113] Kirton SB, Murray CW, Verdonk ML, Taylor RD. Prediction of binding modes for ligands in the cytochromes P450 and other heme-containing proteins. Proteins. 2005;**58**(4):836-844

[114] Doman TN, McGovern SL, Witherbee BJ, Kasten TP, Kurumbail R, Stallings WC, et al. Molecular docking and high-throughput screening for novel inhibitors of protein tyrosine phosphatase-1B. Journal of Medicinal Chemistry. 2002;**45**(11):2213-2221

[115] Shoichet BK, Leach AR, Kuntz ID. Ligand solvation in molecular docking. Proteins. 1999;**34**(1):4-16

[116] Lorber DM, Shoichet BK. Flexible ligand docking using conformational ensembles. Protein Science. 1998;**7**(4):938-950

[117] Freymann DM, Wenck MA, Engel JC, Feng J, Focia PJ, Eakin AE, et al. Efficient identification of inhibitors targeting the closed active site conformation of the HPRT from *Trypanosoma cruzi*. Chemistry & Biology. 2000;7(12):957-968

[118] Su AI, Lorber DM, Weston GS, Baase WA, Matthews BW, Shoichet BK. Docking molecules by families to increase the diversity of hits in database screens: Computational strategy and experimental evaluation. Proteins. 2001;**42**(2):279-293

[119] Gschwend DA, Kuntz ID. Orientational sampling and rigid-body minimization in molecular docking revisited: On-the-fly optimization and degeneracy removal. Journal of Computer-Aided Molecular Design. 1996;**10**(2):123-132

[120] Krovat EM, Steindl T, Langer T. Recent advances in docking and scoring. Journal of Computer-Aided Molecular Design. 2005;**19**:93-102

[121] Kontoyianni M, Sokol GS, McClellan LM. Evaluation of library ranking efficacy in virtual screening. Journal of Computational Chemistry. 2005;**26**:11-22

[122] Kirkpatrick P. Gliding to success. Nature Reviews Drug Discovery. 2004;**3**:299-303

[123] Halgren TA, Murphy RB, Friesner RA, Beard HS, Frye LL, Pollard WT, et al. Glide: A new approach for rapid, accurate docking and scoring. 2. Enrichment factors in database screening. Journal of Msedicinal Chemistry. 2004;**47**:1750-1759

[124] Friesner RA, Banks JL, Murphy RB, Halgren TA, Klicic JJ, Mainz DT, et al. Glide: A new approach for rapid, accurate docking and scoring. 1. Method and assessment of docking accuracy. Journal of Medicinal Chemistry. 2004;**47**:1739-1749

[125] Klon AE, Glick M, Davies JW. Application of machine learning to improve the results of high-throughput docking against the HIV-1 protease. Journal of Chemical Information and Computer Sciences. 2004;**44**:2216-2224

[126] Ruddat VC, Mogul R, Chorny I, Chen C, Perrin N, Whitman S, et al. Tryptophan 500 and Arginine 707 define product and substrate active site binding in soybean lipoxygenase-1. Biochemistry. 2004;**43**:13063-13071

[127] Kellenberger E, Rodrigo J, Muller P, Rognan D. Comparative evaluation of eight docking tools for docking and virtual screening accuracy. Proteins. 2004;**57**:225-242

[128] Perola E, Walters WP, Charifson PS. A detailed comparison of current docking and scoring methods on systems of pharmaceutical relevance. Proteins. 2004;**56**:235-249

[129] Klon AE, Glick M, Thoma M, Acklin P, Davies JW. Finding more needles in the haystack: A simple and efficient method for improving high throughput docking results. Journal of Medicinal Chemistry. 2004;**47**:2743-2749

[130] Bytheway I, Cochran S. Validation of molecular docking calculations involving FGF-1 and FGF-2. Journal of Medicinal Chemistry. 2004;**47**:1683-1693

[131] Kontoyianni M, McClellan LM, Sokol GS. Evaluation of docking performance: Comparative data on docking algorithms. Journal of Medicinal Chemistry. 2004;**47**:558-565

[132] Schulz-Gasch T, Stahl M. Binding site characteristics in structure-based virtual screening: Evaluation of current docking tools. Journal of Molecular Modeling. 2003;**9**:47-57

[133] Wu TYH, Wagner KW, Bursulaya B, Schultz PG, Deveraux QL. Development and characterizationof nonpeptidic

small molecule inhibitors of the XIAP/ caspase-3 interaction. Chemistry and Biology. 2003;**10**:759-767

[134] Kuo GH, Prouty C, DeAngelis A, Shen L, O'Neill DJ, Shah C, et al. Synthesis and discovery of macrocyclic polyoxygenated bis-7-azaindolylmaleimides as a novel series of potent and highly selective glycogen synthase kinase-3β inhibitors. Journal of Medicinal Chemistry. 2003;**46**:4021-4031

[135] Nilsson JW, Kvarnstrom I, Musil D, Nilsson I, Samulesson B. Synthesis and SAR of thrombin inhibitors incorporating a novel 4-amino-morpholinone scaffold: Analysis of x-ray crystal structure of enzyme inhibitor complex. Journal of Medicinal Chemistry. 2003;**46**:3985-4001

[136] Bjerrum EJ, Kristensen AS, Pickering DS, Greenwood JR, Nielsen B, Liljefors T, et al. Design, synthesis, and pharmacology of a highly subtype-selective GluR1/2 agonist, (RS)-2-amino-3-(4-chloro-3-hydroxy-5-isoxazolyl) propionic acid (Cl-HIBO). Journal of Medicinal Chemistry. 2003;**46**:2246-2249

[137] Brehm L, Greenwood JR, Hansen KB, Nielsen B, Egebjerg J, Stensbol TB, et al. (S)-2-amino-3-(3-hydroxy-7,8-dihydro-6H- cyclohepta[d] isoxazol-4-yl)propionic acid, a potent and selective agonist at the GluR5 subtype of ionotropic glutamate receptors. Synthesis, modeling, and molecular pharmacology. Journal of Medicinal Chemistry. 2003;**46**:1350-1358

[138] Thorstensson F, Kvarnstrom I, Musil D, Nilsson I, Samuelsson B. Synthesis of novel thrombin inhibitors. Use of ring-closing metathesis reactions for synthesis of P2 cyclopentene- and cyclohexenedicarboxylic acid derivatives. Journal of Medicinal Chemistry. 2003;**46**:1165-1179

[139] Bunch L, Liljefors T, Greenwood JR, Frydenvang K, Brauner-Osborne H, Krogsgaard-Larsen P, et al. The Journal of Organic Chemistry. 2003;**68**:1489-1495

[140] Raies AB, Bajic VB. In silico toxicology: Computational methods for the prediction of chemical toxicity. Wiley Interdisciplinary Reviews: Computational Molecular Science. 2016;**6**(April):147-172. DOI: 10.1002/wcms.1240

[141] Devillers J. Methods for building QSARs. Methods in Molecular Biology. 2013:**930**:3-27

[142] Parthasarathi R, Dhawan A. In silico approaches for predictive toxicology. In: In Vitro Toxicology. Academic Press. 2018:91-109. DOI: 10.1016/B978-0-12-804667-8.00005-5

[143] Sachdev K, Gupta MK. A comprehensive review of computational techniques for the prediction of drug side effects. Drug Development Research. 2020;**81**(6):650-670. DOI: 10.1002/ddr.21669

[144] Proschak E, Stark H, Merk D. Polypharmacology by design: A medicinal chemist's perspective on multitargeting compounds [review-article]. Journal of Medicinal Chemistry. 2019;**62**(2):420-444. DOI: 10.1021/acs.jmedchem.8b00760

[145] Lavecchia A, Cerchia C. In silico methods to address polypharmacology: Current status, applications and future perspectives. Drug Discovery Today. 2016;**21**(2):288-298. DOI: 10.1016/j.drudis.2015.12.007

[146] Achenbach J, Tiikkainen P, Franke L, Proschak E. Computational tools for polypharmacology and repurposing. Future Medicinal Chemistry. 2011;**3**(8):961-968. DOI: 10.4155/fmc.11.62

[147] Chaudhari R, Tan Z, Huang B, Zhang S. Computational polypharmacology: A new paradigm for drug discovery. Expert Opinion on Drug Discovery. 2017;**12**(3):279-291. DOI: 10.1080/17460441.2017.1280024

[148] Rastelli G, Pinzi L. Computational polypharmacology comes of age. Frontiers in Pharmacology. 2015;**6**(Jul): 1-4. DOI: 10.3389/fphar.2015.00157

[149] Anighoro A, Bajorath J, Rastelli G. Polypharmacology: Challenges and opportunities in drug discovery department of life science informatics, B-IT, LIMES program unit chemical biology and medicinal. Journal of Medicinal Chemistry. 2014;**57**(19):7874-7887

[150] Capdeville R, Buchdunger E, Zimmermann J, Matter A. Glivec (ST1571, imatinib), a rationally developed, targeted anticancer drug. Nature Reviews Drug Discovery. 2002;**1**(7):493-502. DOI: 10.1038/nrd839

[151] Chaudhari R, Fong LW, Tan Z, Huang B, Zhang S. An up-to-date overview of computational polypharmacology in modern drug discovery. Expert Opinion on Drug Discovery. 2020;**15**(9):1025-1044. DOI: 10.1080/17460441.2020.1767063

[152] Medina-Franco JL, Martinez-Mayorga K, Fernández-de Gortari E, Kirchmair J, Bajorath J. Rationality over fashion and hype in drug design. F1000Research. 2021;**10**(397):397

[153] McInnes G, Sharo AG, Koleske ML, Brown JE, Norstad M, Adhikari AN, et al. Opportunities and challenges for the computational interpretation of rare variation in clinically important genes. The American Journal of Human Genetics. 2021;**108**:535-548

[154] Gautam P, Pal MK, Chaudhry V. In silico drug repurposing for MDR bacteria: Opportunities and challenges. In: In Silico Drug Design. Academic Press. 2019. pp. 781-799

[155] Marshall BM, Levy SB. Food animals and antimicrobials: Impacts on human health. Clinical Microbiology Reviews. 2011;**24**(4):718-733

[156] Makhouri FR, Ghasemi JB. In silico studies in drug research against neurodegenerative diseases. Current Neuropharmacology. 2018;**16**:664-725

[157] Baig MH, Ahmad K, Rabbani G, Danishuddin M, Choi I. Computer aided drug design and its application to the development of potential drugs for neurodegenerative disorders. Current Neuropharmacology. 2018;**16**(6):740-748

[158] Verma S, Pathak RK. Discovery and optimization of lead molecules in drug designing. Bioinformatics Methods and Applications. Academic Press. 2022:253-267

[159] Wlodawer A, Vondrasek J. Inhibitors of HIV-1 protease: A major success of structure-assisted drug design. Annual Review of Biophysics and Biomolecular Structure. 1998;**27**:249-284

[160] Anderson AC. The process of structure-based drug design. Chemistry & Biology. 2003;**10**:787-797

[161] Douglas B, Kitchen DB, Decornez HY, Furr JR, Bajorath J. Docking and scoring in virtual screening for drug discovery: Methods and applications. Nature Reviews Drug Discovery. 2004;**3**:935-949

[162] Chen D, Martin ZS, Soto C, Schein CH. Computational selection of inhibitors of Abeta aggregation and neuronal toxicity. Bioorganic

& Medicinal Chemistry. 2009;**17**(14):5189-5197

[163] Cheatham TE, Young MA. Molecular dynamics simulation of nucleic acids: Successes, limitations, and promise. Biopolymers. 2001;**56**(4):232-256

[164] De Paulis T. Drug evaluation: Prx-00023, a selective 5-ht1a receptor agonist for depression. Current Opinion in Investigational Drugs. 2007;**8**:78-86

Chapter 4

Molecular Docking in the Study of Ligand-Protein Recognition: An Overview

Iqbal Azad

Abstract

Molecular docking is a bioinformatics-based theoretical simulation strategy. It is employed to study ligand-protein interaction profiles and predict their binding conformers and affinity through computational tools. Since the 1980s, computational tools have been used in the drug discovery process. The initial molecular modeling approaches available at the time focused on a rigid view of the ligand-protein interaction due to the limited computational capabilities. The advancement of hardware technology has made it possible to simulate the dynamic character of the ligand-protein interactions throughout time. The current chapter deals with an outline of the progression of structure-based drug discovery methodologies in the investigation of the ligand-protein interaction profiles from static to improved molecular docking strategies.

Keywords: Molecular docking, AutoDock, Vina, AutoDockFR, iGEMDOCK, Drug discovery process, Virtual screening

1. Introduction

Docking tools have simplified the study of interactions between drug molecules and receptor proteins, DNA, or biological molecules [1]. These interactions take place covalently. Furthermore, critical molecular mechanisms, ligand binding approaches, and factors influencing the ligand-protein interaction profile can be estimated with the help of the docking results [2, 3]. Docking suites can be used to calculate the binding energies associated with the most stable conformation of drug-receptor interactions (**Figure 1**) [4, 5].

2. Types of docking

In 1982, Kuntz et al. developed the first molecular docking algorithm through the estimation of the released binding energy [6, 7]. Docking evaluations are performed to regulate the interaction profile between the ligand and target and to search for the most suitable conformation of the ligand in the complex. Empirical scoring functions are also explored, which transform binding energy into the docking score [8]. There are numerous free online tools available to generate 3D ligand and target interaction

IntechOpen

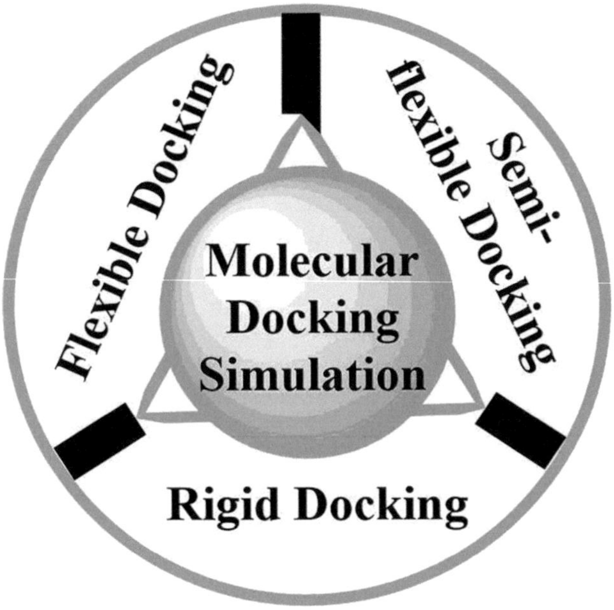

Figure 1.
General modes of molecular docking simulation.

profiles, such as Biovia DSV, Pymol, Chimera, Rasmol, SwissPDB viewer, etc. Docking is broadly classified into three classes, discussed below:

2.1 Flexible docking

In flexible docking, the side chains of the protein and ligand are kept flexible. The general principle of flexible docking is based on the induced-fit hypothesis offered by Daniel Koshland in 1958 [9]. As a result, it is also known as "induced-fit docking," in which the binding energies of various conformations of the proposed ligand are calculated at protein or receptor pockets [10, 11]. Furthermore, the target chain should be flexible enough to combine with the conformational modifications of the receptor and ligand. Various altered possible conformations of the ligand can be predicted, which makes it the most accepted and accurate technique, but it is time-consuming and costly at the same time [12].

2.2 Semi-flexible docking

In this approach, the ligand molecule is the only flexible element while the protein is rigid [13]. In addition to the six translational and rotational degrees of freedom, the conformational degrees of freedom of the ligand are also tested [14]. These approaches assume that a protein's fixed conformation is capable of recognizing the ligands to be docked. As previously stated, this assumption is not always validated [15].

2.3 Rigid docking

In rigid docking, the main geometry of the target and ligand is retained and frozen during docking analysis [16]. The basis of this type of docking analysis is the 'Lock and

Key' hypothesis, proposed by Emil Fischer in 1894 [17]. Thus, it is defined as lock and key docking, which also leads to several problems. The analysis of ligand-target docking is very significant for observing drug-target interaction, but a problem is associated with it when the ligand is docked at the pocket site of a receptor protein. Due to the rigid structure of both, observation of interactions becomes very challenging and the most suitable confirmation of ligand is not easily obtained [18]. Sometimes ligands do not enter the pocket site of a protein, leading to weak interactions that are not enough to show satisfactory results. Internal flexibility is necessary for good docking interaction. In various cases, the structural modifications that are essential for binding are negligible in rigid docking. Rigid docking is only enough to observe the interaction [11]. Some other benefits of rigid docking are its simplicity and a short period of run time.

3. Docking interactions

Docking is performed to establish the most suitable interaction profile for a ligand inside the target protein. It is also employed to estimate the energy evolved during the interaction between the ligand and protein [19]. Various forces influence docking interactions. The total energy released during these interactions is calculated through the empirical formula and displayed in the form of total binding energy [11, 18]. Based on the different forces, docking interactions are categorized as electro-dynamic forces (like van der Waals), electrostatic forces (charge-charge, dipole-dipole, and charge-dipole), steric forces (observed between closer molecules and influence the reactivity as well as the chemical reactivity), solvent-related forces (occurring due to interaction among the solvent and protein/ligand) and conformational modifications in the ligand) [20].

4. Types of energies

The preliminary objective of docking analysis is to obtain the best conformation of the drug during the drug-receptor interactions in support of the lowest binding free energy [21]. Molecular docking tools frequently calculate the scoring functions to evaluate the binding energies of drug-receptor interactions [11]. The resultant binding energy (ΔG bind) is calculated in the form of a combination of different energies such as H-bond, torsional free, electrostatic, unbound system's desolation, total internal, dispersion, and repulsion, etc. The dissociation constant (K_d) is used to signify the binding energy in terms of Gibbs' free energy (ΔG) [22]. The predication of drug-receptor binding depends on the some factors such as intermolecular interactions, desolation, and entropic effects. Upon increasing the estimation of the physiochemical parameters, the accuracy of the scoring function is also increased [23].

An example of a scoring function is as follows:

The empirical scoring function of any docking program.

$$\text{Fitness} = \text{vdW} + \text{H bond} + \text{Elec.}$$

Binding Energy.

$$\Delta G_{\text{bind}} = \Delta G_{\text{vdw}} + \Delta G_{\text{hbond}} + \Delta G_{\text{elect}} + \Delta G_{\text{conform}} + \Delta G_{\text{tor}} + \Delta G_{\text{sol}} \quad (1)$$

5. Docking algorithms

The docking algorithms display a new dimension to evaluating the interaction profile of the ligand-receptor complex [24]. It calculates all possible conformations of the ligand under investigation during the interaction with the receptor. It also delivers the most suitable conformational pose with minimum binding energy [24, 25]. The most common algorithms apply for various docking evaluations (Flexible, Semi-flexible, and Rigid Docking) are (**Figure 2**):

5.1 Flexible docking with single protein conformation

5.1.1 Side-chain flexibility docking

The side-chain flexibility docking approach introduces different conformations for various protein side-chains [26]. This is usually accomplished by utilizing rotamer library databases. Various docking approaches like GOLD use their search engine to sample some degrees of freedom. Large conformational fluctuations of the protein are ignored by these approaches due to side-chain flexibility [27].

5.2 Soft docking

In 1991, Jiang and Kim first described the soft docking strategy, which is based on the understanding of protein flexibility [28]. The VdW revulsion is also working in force field scoring functions because it reduces collisions and allows for more compact ligand-protein packing. In this method, an induced fit is recreated. As a drawback, this method can only simulate faint protein motions, which can lead to erroneous poses [24].

5.3 Flexible docking with multiple protein conformations

For the same target, multiple experimental structures may be offered [29]. Furthermore, computational approaches such as Monte Carlo or Molecular Dynamics

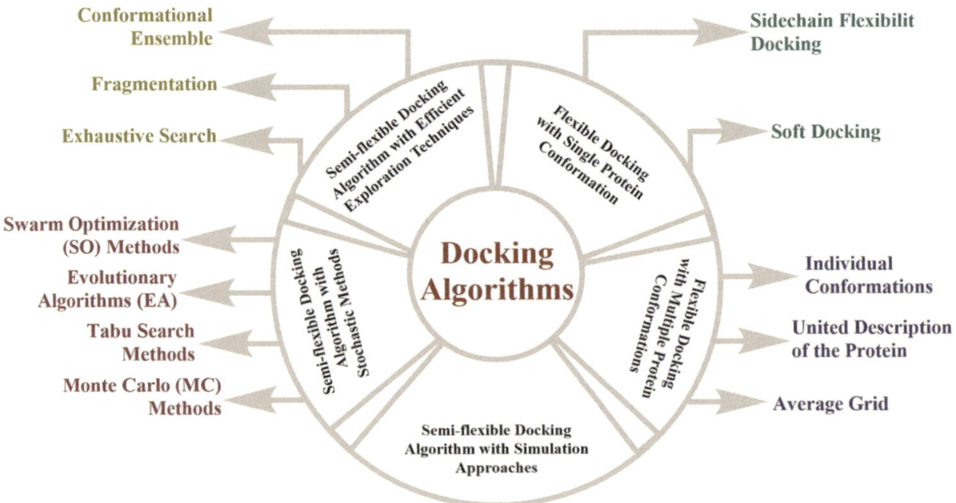

Figure 2.
Various docking algorithms.

simulations can be used to obtain an ensemble of protein conformations [30]. The goal behind multiple protein conformation docking is to consider all of the potential configurations by employing various strategies:

5.3.1 Individual conformations

The target structures are viewed as conformations that could be attached to the ligand. Therefore, several docking scores are undertaken, assessing the ligands on all of the target conformations [31]. Furthermore, to filter the structures, an initial standard to evaluate the presentation of distinct target structures in a docking investigation was also performed in individual conformations [32, 33].

5.3.2 United description of the protein

The structures are utilized to build the best-performing "chimaeras" protein instead of collapsing into an average grid [34]. Like FlexE, it selects structurally conserved areas from the ensemble's structures to build a rigid configuration. This section is attached to the ensemble's flexible portions in a combinatorial method, resulting in a pool of "chimaeras" that can be docked [35].

5.3.3 Average grid

The ensemble's structures are combined to form a typical solitary grid [36].

5.4 Semi-flexible docking algorithm with simulation approaches

A well-known model of this class is molecular dynamics. This approach defines a system's temporal evolution [37]. The molecular dynamics unit provides a more detailed explanation [38]. Energy-saving strategies are also included in this category, but these strategies are rarely utilized as standalone search engines [39]. Energy minimization is a local optimization approach for obtaining a system with certain potential energy [40].

5.5 Semi-flexible docking algorithm with stochastic methods

In this approach, the values of the degrees of freedom of a system are changed randomly rather than systematically like in stochastic algorithms [41]. The speed of these procedures is beneficial, as they might potentially locate the best answer very quickly. The main disadvantage of this approach is that it does not confirm a comprehensive investigation of the conformational space, which denotes the actual solution, which may be overlooked. Increase the number of iterations of the method to partially solve the lack of convergence. The following are the most well-known stochastic algorithms [42]:

5.5.1 Swarm optimization (SO) methods

Several swarm optimization approaches are based on the behavior of swarms [43]. The knowledge supplied by previously sampling good poses guides the sample of a ligand's degrees of freedom. PLANTS use an Ant Colony Optimization (ACO) algorithm, which simulates the behavior of ants, and uses pheromones to find the quickest way to a food position [44]. Each degree of freedom is coupled with a pheromone in this system. Successful ants contribute to pheromone deposition, while virtual ants choose conformations based on pheromone values.

5.5.2 Evolutionary algorithms (EA)

The most prominent evolutionary algorithms are genetic algorithms (GAs), which are based on the idea of biological evolution [45]. The genes, chromosomes, mutations, and crossover concepts are all taken from biology. Genes are represented in the form of the degrees of freedom as well as ligand conformation, which is defined by a chromosome that is awarded a fitness score [46]. Within a population of chromosomes, mutations and crossovers occur, and the chromosomes with greater fitness survive and replace the ones with lower fitness. rDock, PSI-DOCk, AutoDock, and GOLD are the most well-known instances [46–50].

5.5.3 Tabu search methods

Tabu search strategies are used to avoid exploring zones of the conformational/ positional space that have already been explored. At each cycle, random alterations are made to the ligand's degrees of freedom. The previously sampled conformations are recorded, and a new stance is allowed only if it is distinct from any previously investigated pose. This category includes programs like PRO LEADS and PSI-DOCK [47, 51–54].

5.5.4 Monte Carlo (MC) methods

The Metropolis Monte Carlo algorithm, which presents a recognized measure in the development of docking exploration, is the basis for Monte Carlo approaches [55]. Each repetition of the algorithm involves a casual adjustment of the degrees of freedom of the ligand. The Metropolis algorithm in its basic form, although it is implemented in a variety of ways in docking software, AutoDock Vina, MCDOCK, QXP, ICM, and AutoDock [30, 42, 44, 56].

5.6 Semi-flexible docking algorithm with efficient exploration techniques

In an efficient exploration, a collection of findings is associated with each degree of freedom, and all the values of each coordinate are examined in a combinatorial manner [56]. These approaches are classified into the following categories:

5.6.1 Conformational ensemble

Rigid docking approaches can easily be supplemented with a certain amount of flexibility. If an ensemble of previously produced ligand conformers is docked to the target using a conformational variation approach on the ligand complement, an example is MS-DOCK [57].

5.6.2 Fragmentation

DesJarlais et al. in 1986 described an approach to fragmentation of the ligand. The first application of ligand flexibility in docking was the hard docking of fragments into the reaction site and the subsequent connecting of the fragments [58]. Partial flexibility is achieved at the junctions among the fragments in this manner. Additional approaches, known as incremental building, initially dock one fragment and then add the rest, one by one. FlexX [59] and Hammerhead [60] are two approaches that use fragmentation [61].

5.6.3 Exhaustive search

Exhaustive exploration is an efficient method in austere intelligence, as it examines all of the ligands' rotatable bonds systematically. To limit the search space and avoid a combinatorial explosion, several limitations and termination criteria are usually defined. The software Glide's docking pipeline [62, 63] includes an exhaustive search stage.

6. Some common docking software

6.1 AutoDock

AutoDock is an open-source and automated docking package introduced by the Molecular Graphics Lab, Scripps Research Institute, La Jolla, CA 92037, USA. It is effectively applied to the calculation of the binding sphere of biological macromolecules like proteins and enzymes, as well as ligands (small molecules) [25]. The AutoDock docking suite offers the minimum binding energy of interaction obtained between the ligand and the receptor protein. The binding energy calculation is based on the formula offered in the form of the scoring function. Using the Lamarckian genetic algorithm (LGA), the AutoDock scoring function is established on the AMBER force field as well as through linear regression analysis [64]. It deals with reinforcing docking evaluation for ligands through almost zero to ten flexible bonds. The default settings of AutoDock are tremendously effective and are commonly applied to search for the interaction profile of a drug candidate. Furthermore, it is also extensively used for virtual screening. For each docking, the AutoDock is performed for a considerable duration to provide frequently docked conformations of the ligand concerning a receptor protein [65]. Examples: drug-receptor docking; protein-protein docking; molecule optimization; analysis oscillating from structure-based drug design; validation of the action mechanism of drug molecules; etc.

6.2 Handling tips of AutoDock

AutoDock tools offer multiple approaches for docking simulation, such as alternating from simple docking to advanced docking procedures [66]. The successful run of AutoDock requires four different files, such as ligand coordinates, target coordinates, grid parameters, and docking parameters [67, 68]. These files are prepared with the help of AutoDock Tools (ADT)/MGL Tools and their preparatory procedures are as follows:

6.3 Preparation ligand coordinate file

AutoDock accepts PDB or mol2 files as an input. In the novel compound, the first three-dimensional (3D) structure of the compound is prepared. The two-dimensional

(2D) structure of the proposed compound can be prepared with the help of ChemDraw or ChemDoodle (https://web.chemdoodle.com/demos/sketcher/) and saved as a SMILES file. The SMILES file is pasted into the online CORINA Classic service (https://www.mn-am.com/online_demos/corina_demo) to prepare meals or. pdb files, but it needs further structural optimization through a suitable method such as Merck Molecular Force Field (MMFF). On the other hand, for simple preparation to optimize 3D structures, the online molsoft (https://www.molsoft.com/2dto3d.html) is recommended. It can prepare 2D as well as 3D structures in a single place. During the conversion of a 2D structure into 3D, it automatically optimizes the structure through MMFF. It has been found that the most accurate, optimized structure can be offered by DFT, but MMFF is still useful for an organic molecule. If the proposed compound has a known structure, then its crystalline 3D structure can be obtained from PubChem (https://pubchem.ncbi.nlm.nih.gov)and ChemSpider (http://www.che mspider.com/), etc. The coordinate setting of proposed compounds needs the addition of hydrogen atoms that are included in the 3D structure [69]. The proposed compound's open 3D structure is selected as a ligand in ADT, and the 'edit' button is clicked to add polar hydrogens, Gasteiger charge, number of torsions, and detect root. At this moment, the ligand will be visible on the screen in which aromatic carbons appear green and another fragment looks red. Now click 'ok' and save it as a ligand pdbqt file.

6.4 Preparation of target coordinate file

ADT also requires preparing the coordinates of a biological macromolecule such as a protein or enzyme. The PDB file of the receptor can be downloaded from the Protein Data Bank (www.pdb.org), the Cambridge Crystallographic Database (ccdc.cam.ac.uk), etc. To generate the target coordinate file, all hydrogen atoms, need to be added. The 3D coordinates of the target can be taken from the PDB, and it requires the removal of water, ligands, cofactors, ions, etc. Click on 'Edit' to incorporate polar hydrogen, Kollman charge, Marge nonpolar hydrogen, and macromolecules are saved as target pdbqt.

6.5 Preparation grid parameter file

ADT needs a pdbqt file to prepare the grid parameter file (gpf). In a new window to set the grid, click on Grid > Macromolecule > Open and open the target pdbqt file by macromolecule. Similarly, click on Grid > Set map type > Open and open the ligand pdbqt file of the proposed small molecule or ligand, and then set the grid map, grid size, as well as grid center in x, y, and z-direction by clicking on "grid > Grid box". After that, the output file can be saved as a gpf file.

6.6 Preparation docking parameter file

For the preparation of the docking parameter file (dpf), click on Docking > Macromolecule > Set rigid filament > Open in the ADT window to open the target PDBQT. Similarly, ligand pdbqt can also be opened by clicking on Docking > Ligand > Open. Then, set the algorithm by clicking on Docking > Search Parameters > Genetic algorithm and setting docking parameters. Finally, click on Docking > Output > Lararckian GA and save it as a dpf file. Then ADT is ready to run. Firstly, it runs. It required a proper time and needed the grid parameter file as well as a docking parameter file.

6.7 Analysis of docking result

ADT also offers to evaluate docking interactions and binding energies of a minimum of ten conformations along with a docking inhibition constant (K_a). By selecting Analyze > Docking > Open, you may view the findings by opening the dlg file. A popup will open, click "OK" and then further click Analyze > Conformation > Play > & > Show info.

The AutoDock scoring function can be calculated based on the following formula:

$$\text{Free binding energy} = \text{Final intermolecular energy} + \text{Final total internal energy} \\ + \text{Torsional free energy - Unbound system's energy.}$$

Where, total energy of van der Waal energy, hydrogen bond energy, electrostatic energy and dissolved energy equals to final intermolecular energy.

7. AutoDock Vina

AutoDock Vina was established by Oleg Trott in the Molecular Graphics Lab at the Scripps Research Institute in 2010 [70]. It is a relatively new, freely available tool for molecular docking, drug discovery, and virtual screening. It also offers high performance, multi-core proficiency, greater accuracy, and a simple handling protocol. Vina itself predicts the grid maps and clusters. Vina considerably enhances the accuracy of the interaction mode calculations as associated with AutoDock. Vina has been found to predict more accurate results as compared to other tools [71].

7.1 Handling tips of AutoDock Vina

The input and output files of Vina are pdbqt. It is essential to prepare the ligand as well as the target coordinate file in pdbqt format. Both coordinate files are prepared similarly as in AutoDock. Vina does not require a grid parameter file and a docking parameter file [72]. Additionally, it requires a text configuration file. Complete handling of AutoDock Vina is discussed below.

7.2 Preparation of configuration file

A new window of ADT is opened after the preparation of the ligand and target coordinate file. Click on Grid > Macromolecule > Open and open the target pdbqt file. Click "YES" to save the present modifications in the folder, and then press "OK" to receive them. Sometimes a warning window is also opened if there are minor indiscretions in charge. Ignore it by pressing "OK."

Then, click Grid > Set map types > Open and open the ligand pdbqt file. The grid map, grid size, and grid center of the analysis space are then described in a new window that is opened by selecting Grid > Grid box. To begin the box built on the ligand, click Center > Center on the ligand. Here, thumbnails are available for the manual changes in the values of grid size and center, along with other options. Press file > close to save the current after adjusting the grid's size and center. To complete the setup, select Docking > Output > Vina Configuration and click "SAVE" to provide a text configuration file with the default name of config.txt.

7.3 Run AutoDock Vina

The default setting of AutoDock Vina is not enough to accurately evaluate the interaction profile and binding energies. Vina offers a factor known as exhaustiveness to adjust the computer-aided strength utilized during a docking analysis. In Vina, the default value of exhaustiveness is 8. For greater accuracy, the default value of exhaustiveness is changed and set to about 24. It will provide more accurate docking findings. The most well-known way to run Vina is via ADT. ADT offers to click "run" to run AutoDock Vina. Open a window to start the route of the Vina executable file by pressing the browse option, and then press the launch button to operate the Vina. The second path is through the command line. Open a terminal window and modify the directory that encompasses the coordinate files as well as the configuration file. The command line is edited to adjust the values of exhaustiveness (like: /Vina–config config.txt-exhaustiveness = 24). This command accepts that the AutoDock Vina executable Vina is also found in a similar directory.

7.4 Analysis of Vina docking result

ADT also offers the ability to visualize the outcomes of docking from AutoDock Vina. Open a new ADT window and select the working directory. Analyze > Docking > Open the AutoDock Vina result and select the output file obtained from step II. Then select the default single molecule with numerous conformations followed by pressing "OK" to visualize the coordinates for all docked outcomes through arrow keys. To visualize the target coordinate file, select Analyze > Macromolecule > Open and open the target pdbqt file. Similarly, open the ligand coordinate file by clicking on File > Read molecule > Open and open the ligand pdbqt file to read the crystallographic location of the ligand. It offers the ability to evaluate the ligand as well as docked conformation. Select Analyze > Docking > Show interactions to examine the ligand-target complex's interaction profile.

The estimated scoring function of AutoDock Vina is based on the following formula:

$$\Delta G\ (\text{binding}) = \Delta G\ (\text{vdW}) + \Delta G\ (\text{H bond}) + \Delta G\ (\text{Elec.}) + \Delta G\ (\text{E desolv.}) \quad (2)$$

Where ΔG denotes Gibbs' free energy, ΔG (vdW) denotes van der Waal's free energy, and ΔG (H bond) denotes hydrogen bond free energy. ΔG (Elec.) stands for electrostatic free energy; ΔG (E dissolv.) stands for dissolved free energy. Torsional free energy is denoted by the symbol ΔG (tors).

8. AutoDock FR

AutoDock FR (ADFR: AutoDock for Flexible Receptors) was developed by Dr. Pradeep Anand Ravindranath in the Integrative Structural and Computational Biology Lab at the Scripps Research Institute in 2015. The ADFR is a newly designed docking tool built for the AutoDock scoring function. The ADFR was deliberately designed to study the interaction of small flexible ligands with the target protein [69, 73]. It offers preparation of side-chains of target proteins flexibly to simulate induced-fit without the knowledge of the side-chain conformational alterations [73]. The ADFR regulates up to 14 targets with side-chain flexibility. The proficient growth rate of docking realization is more than 50%. On the cross, docking is investigated along with up to 12 flexible receptor side-chains. The ADFR displays superior results as compared to AutoDock Vina. Vina requires uncontrolled run time for docking by increasing the number of flexible receptor side chains. On the other hand, ADFR requires linear run time [73].

8.1 Handling tips of AutoDockFR

The input format of ADFR is pdbqt format. ADFR requires the preparation of coordinate files of ligand and target. Coordinate files are prepared with the help of ADT. To perform docking through ADFR also requires the generation of affinity maps and translational points that are probable ligand binding areas. The step-by-step handling protocol of ADFR is discussed below.

8.2 Prepare affinity maps and translational points

Open a new ADFR window, select the receptor PDBQT > Open, and upload the target coordinate file in pdbqt format to run the docking analysis. Similarly, the ligand pdbqt file is uploaded by selecting Open under ligand PDBQT. Then press the box entire ligand button to surround the ligand with a docking box or grid box, followed by clicking on the center view of the docking box to center the docking position. In the docking box, along with ligand, amino acid residues can also be labeled by clicking on "show receptor residue labels." ADFR is the only tool to select the amino acid residue up to 14 at a time with a single click. To select the amino acid residues for docking investigation, click on flexible residues and select the amino acids from the list. The selected side chains of the amino acid are presented as orange balls-sticks and the other portions remain the same. Then click the green checkmark.

For the prediction of binding pockets, click on the 'compute pockets' button. Auto Site recognizes multiple pockets in the docking box and selects those at which the actual ligand is found in higher volume. These binding pocket fill-points appear as a green mesh, denoted as translational points. If the binding pocket fills-points button is green, then generating maps is supported. To generate affinity maps, press the Generate maps button and save the maps as a zip file in the working folder.

8.3 Run ADFR

Open the command window, adjust the working directory, and type the following windows command to run the ADFR: "c:\Program Files\MGL Tools 2-latest\adfr.bat" random pdbqt -m generate.zip -r ligand pdbqt -job Name Result –seed −1. To visualize the docking result, a visualization tool like Biovia DSV is used to generate the interaction profile of the ligand-target complex.

9. iGEMDOCK

The iGEMDOCK tool was established by the Institute of Bioinformatics at National Chiao Tung University, Taiwan for docking, drug design, screening, and post-screening analysis. It is an automatic multipurpose graphical package [74]. For docking evaluation on the iGEMDOCK, initially prepare the coordinate files of the ligand as well as the target. Coordinate files are prepared similarly as in AutoDock by adding torsions, bond orders, hydrogen atoms, and charges. These parameters are assigned to both the ligand and the target. The input and output files of the iGEMDOCK are PDB and Mol. IGEMDOCK automatically selects the most suitable conformation of the ligand and gives the total binding energy [74]. The iGEMDOCK scores are calculated using an empirical formula or fitness score, denoted as.

Van der Waal energy + Hydrogen bond energy + Electro-statistic energy equals fitness score.

During the docking evaluation, the estimation of target binding sites and structure optimization are very significant. The hydrogen bonds found in the docked complex strongly impact the scoring function. This possibility reduces the number of suspected H bonds significantly. Additionally, internal H bonds, as well as internal electrostatic interaction, are predicted as sp2-sp2 torsions from the interaction complex. The iGEMDOCK works, since the generic evolutionary method (GA), provides three effective docking methods, *viz.,* standard docking, stable docking, and accurate docking. Accurate docking is a very slow docking protocol and offers a maximum of 80 numbers of runs or generations, 800 population size, 8000 interactions, and 10 numbers of the solution, along with 100-threshold energy. For every single step, torsions, translations, and rotations are verified. For a better result, the hydrophobic, as well as electrostatic preferences are set to 1.00. The iGEMDOCK automatically selects the lowest energy conformation. When the iGEMDOCK calculates unfavorable electrostatic interaction, then a positive energy value is obtained. To rectify this problem, check the docked position and restart; or if the docked pose is closer to the listed ligands, define the RMSD threshold and add an energy penalty (i.e., the 100-energy penalty, 2.00 RMSD threshold, and atom ID (fast) RMSD calculations were set.) In the scoring function, the docking tool resolves and emphasizes the results of its previous search and finds their variations. Then ligand-target docking proceeds and results are obtained in the form of binding affinities (kcal/Mol) and docking run time. The minimum binding energy conformation is automatically selected as the best finding. The overall docking performance of the iGEMDOCK as compared to other docking tools is simple and better.

9.1 Handling tips of iGEMDOCK

The iGEMDOCK is a complete package of automated docking and screening. It is a combination of two main parts; the first part predicts the interaction profile among the ligand-target complex in the 3D structure, while the second part predicts the suitable pose of the ligand-target complex along with post-analysis. The docking evaluation with the iGEMDOCK begins with the preparation of ligand and target protein coordinate files. Both coordinate files are prepared like AutoDock. The iGEMDOCK input and output file formats are mol, mol2, and PDB.

9.2 Target binding site preparation

In the iGEMDOCK operator, a distinct binding site of the target protein/enzyme or complete target structure is selected. If the target's input file contains a natural

Server/Software	Availability	Developer	City/ Country	Web link
AutoDock 4	Free standalone program	The Scripps Research Institute	La Jolla, CA/ US	http://autodock.scripps.edu/
AutoDock Vina	Free standalone program	The Scripps Research Institute	La Jolla, CA/ US	http://vina.scripps.edu/
BioXGEM.iGEMDOCK	Free/open-source platform	BioXGEM Lab. Institute of Bioinformatics National Chiao-Tung University	Hsinchu/ Taiwan	http://gemdock.life.nctu.edu.tw/
DOCK	Free/open-source platform	University of California, San Francisco	San Francisco, California/ USA	http://dock.compbio.ucsf.edu/
GOLD	Commercially available	The Cambridge Crystallographic Data Centre	Cambridge/ USA	https://www.ccdc.cam.ac.uk/solutions/csd-discovery/components/gold/
Glide	Commercially available	Schrödinger, LLC	New York/ USA	https://www.schrodinger.com/glide
BioSolveIT FlexX4	Commercially available	BioSolveIT GmbH	Sankt Augustin/ Germany	https://www.biosolveit.de/FlexX/
SIB Swiss Institute of Bioinformatics	Free webserver	Swiss Institute of Bioinformatics	Lausanne/ Switzerland	http://www.swissadme.ch/
CDOCKER	Commercially available	BIOVIA	San Diego/ California, USA	https://www.3dsbiovia.com/
Pharmer	Free/open-source platform	Department of Computational Biology, University of Pittsburgh	Pittsburgh/ Pennsylvania	http://smoothdock.ccbb.pitt.edu/pharmer/

Table 1.
The server/software of the molecular docking analysis.

physiological ligand, it will automatically determine the target's binding site. To begin docking, upload the target's coordinate file (PDB) by clicking "Prepare binding site > Browse > Open" in the "Protein-ligand docking/screening" window. To select the binding site of the target, click on "By bounded ligand" and then define the binding site center by selecting the available ligand which you want to study. It also offers to set the binding site radius; by default, its value is 8.0 Å. Uncheck the "Retain reference ligand" box, and then click "OK" to save the defined parameter to the chosen binding site. This will delete the physiological ligand. Select "by a current file" to specify the binding sites of the new target protein.

9.3 Ligand preparation

The iGEMDOCK provides two methods for ligand preparation. To begin, for "single ligand," upload the ligand coordinate file (single/many) directly by clicking "Prepare compounds > Ligands > Open" and pressing "OK" at the "docking/screening" window. The iGEMDOCK recommends preparing the ligand coordinate file in mol. It does not assign charges and hydrogen to all of the ligand's atoms. For the "ligand database", the ligand library is also prepared as mol. To upload the list of compounds, click "Prepare compounds," then "import list," "Open," and "OK."

9.4 Run iGEMDOCK

Set the output path before the start of docking evaluation. Set the output path by clicking on the "Set output path". Then choose the desired file and press "OK."

Set the GA Parameters: iGEMDOCK works based on the generic evolutionary method (GA) for docking performance. It automatically calculates the ligand conformation as well as orientation compared to the interaction site of the target. The following default GA parameters are generally recommended: population size: 200; generations: 70; and a number of solutions: 3.

Advanced Options: The iGEMDOCK offers an advanced option for the adjustment of the scoring function, saving/loading configurations, and generating docking poses. It also allows setting the internal energy of the ligand in docking prediction or the addition of certain molecular filters. It automatically produces a configuration file with the name config.dock file in the directory "/bin/". Set up all the parameters in the configuration file and run it with the help of command mode.

Start Docking: After the setting of coordinate files of ligand and target along with output path and docking parameters, press "start docking" and observe the status of the job on the screen. After the completion of docking, a default alert is opened. To close it, click "OK," then press "View docked poses > post-analyze" to visualize the docking poses and the complete binding energy of the docked complex. These docking poses will be saved in the "best_pose" and "fitness.txt" at the output site, respectively (**Table 1**).

10. Use of molecular docking

In the last decade, technologies like high-throughput sequencing and X-ray crystallography have been regularly updated. The crystal structures of large numbers of proteins have been defined. Consequently, the structural and functional significance of biological macromolecules (like proteins and enzymes) has been expanded and many novel drug targets also have been identified [75]. Due to the revolution of computational science in various fields of research, the utilization of virtual screening and molecular docking in DDD has been significantly stimulated. The development of a novel drug is time-consuming, costly, and needs more manpower [76]. Currently, computer-aided technology has become a key tool in DDD. Through molecular docking simulation, the analysis of the mutual interaction of drug and receptor becomes very easy along with high accuracy and boosts the drug development procedure by reducing the time [77].

Reverse molecular docking is a particularly fresh and innovative significant of molecular docking. It precedes the library of small molecules as a key structure to execute molecular docking in the spatial or 3D target database and evaluate the conceivable larger entities to conclude the three-dimensional structure and energy of identical assessment. That is to say, it identifies the most suitable target with minimum binding energy. For that reason, the development of reverse molecular docking provides a new route to discover the suitable target of a drug compound and reveal the drug action mechanism [78].

11. Conclusion

The findings of this chapter demonstrate that docking programs are highly focused on the development of new pharmaceutical compounds using molecular modeling. In this decade, new docking software designs are emphasized. These trends are focused on improving docking accuracy by using more accurate molecular energy calculations without any fitting parameters, such as quantum-chemical methods, implicit solvent models, and new global optimization algorithms that can treat ligand flexibility and protein atom mobility at the same time. Current docking applications are not reliable enough to estimate binding affinity due to the insufficient molecular structure and the inadequacies of the scoring algorithm. However, by including a huge amount of biological data into the scoring function, the present molecular docking technique can be improved. Finally, it is demonstrated that all of the conditions for improving docking accuracy may be met in practice. Furthermore, some expanded sampling strategies are no longer an exclusive methodological exercise but have become accessible to a wide range of research organizations, with real-world applications in drug discovery. Molecular docking, technological advancements, and novel MD computational approaches have all made it possible to simulate increasingly large conformational shifts. By providing a mechanical understanding of binding pathways, the ability to recreate present folding and binding processes can be used to address the long-standing argument regarding "induced-fit" and "conformational selection" binding theories.

Acknowledgements

The authors gratefully acknowledge the R&D wing of Integral University, Lucknow, for their support and guidance.

Conflict of interest

The authors declare no conflict of interest.

Author details

Iqbal Azad
Department of Chemistry, Integral University, Lucknow, UP, India

*Address all correspondence to: iazad@iul.ac.in

References

[1] Chen G, Seukep AJ, Guo M. Recent advances in molecular docking for the research and discovery of potential marine drugs. Marine Drugs. 2020; **18**(11):545-566

[2] Guedes IA, de Magalhães CS, Dardenne LE. Receptor–ligand molecular docking. Biophysical Reviews. 2014;**6**(1):75

[3] Pantsar T, Poso A. Binding affinity via docking: Fact and fiction. Mol A J Synth Chem Nat Prod Chem. 2018; **23**(8):1899-1909

[4] Mazumder M, Ponnan P, Das U, Gourinath S, Khan HA, Yang J, et al. Investigations on binding pattern of kinase inhibitors with PPAR γ: Molecular docking, molecular dynamic simulations, and free energy calculation studies. PPAR Research. 2017;**2017**: 6397836

[5] Ramírez D, Caballero J. Is it reliable to use common molecular docking methods for comparing the binding affinities of enantiomer pairs for their protein target? International Journal of Molecular Sciences. 2016;**17**(4):525-539

[6] Kuntz ID, Blaney JM, Oatley SJ, Langridge R, Ferrin TE. A geometric approach to macromolecule-ligand interactions. Journal of Molecular Biology. 1982;**161**(2):269-288

[7] Ahmed A, Mam B, Sowdhamini R. DEELIG: A deep learning approach to predict protein-ligand binding affinity. Bioinformatics and Biology Insights. 2021;**15**:1-9

[8] Guedes IA, Pereira FSS, Dardenne LE. Empirical scoring functions for structure-based virtual screening: Applications, critical aspects, and challenges. Frontiers in Pharmacology. 2018;**9**:1089

[9] Koshland DE. The key–lock theory and the induced fit theory. Angew Chemie Int Ed English. 1995;**33**(23–24): 2375-2378

[10] Lexa KW, Carlson HA. Protein flexibility in docking and surface mapping. Quarterly Reviews of Biophysics. 2012;**45**(3):301-343

[11] Tripathi A, Bankaitis VA. Molecular docking: From lock and key to combination lock. J Mol Med Clin Appl. 2017;**2**(1). DOI: 10.16966/ 2575-0305.106

[12] Andrusier N, Mashiach E, Nussinov R, Wolfson HJ. Principles of flexible protein-protein docking. Proteins: Structure, Function and Genetics. 2008;**73**(2):271-289

[13] Anderson AC, O'Neil RH, Surti TS, Stroud RM. Approaches to solving the rigid receptor problem by identifying a minimal set of flexible residues during ligand docking. Chemistry & Biology. 2001;**8**(5):445-457

[14] Meng X-Y, Zhang H-X, Mezei M, Cui M. Molecular docking: A powerful approach for structure-based drug discovery. Current Computer-Aided Drug Design. 2011;7(2):146-157

[15] Du X, Li Y, Xia YL, Ai SM, Liang J, Sang P, et al. Insights into protein–ligand interactions: Mechanisms, models, and methods. International Journal of Molecular Sciences. 2016;**17**(2):144-177

[16] Cramer F. Biochemical correctness: Emil Fischer's lock and key hypothesis, a hundred years after — An essay.

Pharmaceutica Acta Helvetiae. 1995; **69**(4):193-203

[17] Salmaso V, Moro S. Bridging molecular docking to molecular dynamics in exploring ligand-protein recognition process: An overview. Frontiers in Pharmacology. 2018;**9**:923

[18] Meng X-Y, Zhang H-X, Mezei M, Cui M. Molecular docking: A powerful approach for structure-based drug discovery. Curr Comput Aided-Drug Des. 2012;**7**(2):146-157

[19] Pinzi L, Rastelli G. Molecular docking: Shifting paradigms in drug discovery. International Journal of Molecular Sciences. 2019;**20**(18):4331

[20] Hetényi C, Van Der Spoel D. Blind docking of drug-sized compounds to proteins with up to a thousand residues. FEBS Letters. 2006;**580**(5):1447-1450

[21] Ferreira LG, Dos Santos RN, Oliva G, Andricopulo AD. Molecular docking and structure-based drug design strategies. Molecules. 2015;**20**(7):13384

[22] Hall R, Dixon T, Dickson A. On calculating free energy differences using ensembles of transition paths. Frontiers in Molecular Biosciences. 2020;**7**:106

[23] Agrawal P, Singh H, Srivastava HK, Singh S, Kishore G, Raghava GPS. Benchmarking of different molecular docking methods for protein-peptide docking. BMC Bioinformatics. 2019;**19**: 426

[24] Torres PHM, Sodero ACR, Jofily P, Silva-Jr FP. Key topics in molecular docking for drug design. International Journal of Molecular Sciences. 2019; **20**(18):4574

[25] Morris GM, Goodsell DS, Halliday RS, Huey R, Hart WE, Belew RK, et al. Automated docking using a Lamarckian genetic algorithm and an empirical binding free energy function. Journal of Computational Chemistry. 1998;**19**(14):1639-1662

[26] Zavodszky MI, Kuhn LA. Side-chain flexibility in protein–ligand binding: The minimal rotation hypothesis. Protein Science. 2005;**14**(4):1104

[27] Miao Z, Cao Y. Quantifying side-chain conformational variations in protein structure. Sci Reports. 2016;**6**(1): 1-10

[28] Jiang F, Kim SH. "Soft docking": Matching of molecular surface cubes. Journal of Molecular Biology. 1991; **219**(1):79-102

[29] Lepore R, Kryshtafovych A, Alahuhta M, Veraszto HA, Bomble YJ, Bufton JC, et al. Target highlights in CASP13: Experimental target structures through the eyes of their authors. Proteins Struct Funct Bioinforma. 2019; **87**(12):1037-1057

[30] Hospital A, Goñi JR, Orozco M, Gelpí JL. Molecular dynamics simulations: Advances and applications. Adv Appl Bioinform Chem. 2015;**8**(1):37

[31] Huang SY, Zou X. Ensemble docking of multiple protein structures: Considering protein structural variations in molecular docking. Proteins. 2007;**66**(2):399-421

[32] Salmaso N, Stevens HE, McNeill J, ElSayed M, Ren Q, Maragnoli ME, et al. Fibroblast growth factor 2 modulates hypothalamic pituitary Axis activity and anxiety behavior through glucocorticoid receptors. Biological Psychiatry. 2016; **80**(6):479-489

[33] Al-Karmalawy AA, Dahab MA, Metwaly AM, Elhady SS, Elkaeed EB, Eissa IH, et al. Molecular docking and

dynamics simulation revealed the potential inhibitory activity of ACEIs against SARS-CoV-2 targeting the hACE2 receptor. Frontiers in Chemistry. 2021;**9**:661230

[34] Seidel R, Blumer M, Chaumel J, Amini S, Dean MN. Endoskeletal mineralization in chimaera and a comparative guide to tessellated cartilage in chondrichthyan fishes (sharks, rays and chimaera). J R Soc Interface. 2020; **17**:20200474

[35] Gallego-Yerga L, Ochoa R, Lans I, Peña-Varas C, Alegría-Arcos M, Cossio P, et al. Application of ensemble pharmacophore-based virtual screening to the discovery of novel antimitotic tubulin inhibitors. Computational and Structural Biotechnology Journal. 2021; **19**:4360-4372

[36] Knegtel RMA, Kuntz ID, Oshiro CM. Molecular docking to ensembles of protein structures. Journal of Molecular Biology. 1997;**266**(2):424-440

[37] Adcock SA, McCammon JA. Molecular dynamics: Survey of methods for simulating the activity of proteins. Chemical Reviews. 2006;**106**(5):1589

[38] Hollingsworth SA, Dror RO. Molecular dynamics simulation for all. Neuron. 2018;**99**(6):1129

[39] Kitchen DB, Decornez H, Furr JR, Bajorath J. Docking and scoring in virtual screening for drug discovery: Methods and applications. Nature Reviews. Drug Discovery. 2004;**3**(11):935-949

[40] Gautam B. Energy Minimization. In: Maia RT, de Moraes Filho Ra, Campos M. editors. Homology Molecular Modeling - Perspectives and Applications. London: IntechOpen; 2020. DOI: 10.5772/intechopen.94809

[41] Araki M, Matsumoto S, Bekker GJ, et al. Exploring ligand binding pathways on proteins using hypersound-accelerated molecular dynamics. Nature Communications. 2021;**12**:2793

[42] Huang SY, Zou X. Advances and challenges in protein-ligand docking. International Journal of Molecular Sciences. 2010;**11**(8):3016-3034

[43] Korb O, Stützle T, Exner TE. PLANTS: Application of ant Colony optimization to structure-based drug design. Lecture Notes in Computer Science. 2006;**4150**:247-258

[44] Katoch S, Chauhan SS, Kumar V. A review on genetic algorithm: Past, present, and future. Multimedia Tools and Applications. 2021;**80**(5):8091-8126

[45] Tessaro F, Tessaro F, Scapozza L, Scapozza L. How 'protein-docking' translates into the new emerging field of docking small molecules to nucleic acids? Molecules. 2020;**25**(12):2749

[46] Xu J, Zhang L, Ye Y, Shan Y, Wan C, Wang J, et al. SNX16 regulates the recycling of E-cadherin through a unique mechanism of coordinated membrane and cargo binding. Structure. 2017;**25**(8): 1251-1263.e5

[47] Pei J, Wang Q, Liu Z, Li Q, Yang K, Lai L. PSI-DOCK: Towards highly efficient and accurate flexible ligand docking. Proteins Struct Funct Bioinforma. 2006;**62**(4):934-946

[48] Jones S, Thornton JM. Prediction of protein-protein interaction sites using patch analysis. Journal of Molecular Biology. 1997;**272**(1):133-143

[49] Yan Y, He J, Feng Y, Lin P, Tao H, Huang SY. Challenges and opportunities of automated protein-protein docking: HDOCK server vs human predictions in

CAPRI rounds 38-46. Proteins Struct Funct Bioinforma. 2020;**88**(8): 1055-1069

[50] Ruiz-Carmona S, Alvarez-Garcia D, Foloppe N, Garmendia-Doval AB, Juhos S, Schmidtke P, et al. rDock: A fast, versatile and open source program for docking ligands to proteins and nucleic acids. PLoS Computational Biology. 2014;**10**(4):e1003571

[51] Verdonk ML, Cole JC, Hartshorn MJ, Murray CW, Taylor RD. Improved protein-ligand docking using GOLD. Proteins: Structure, Function, and Genetics. 2003;**52**(4):609-623

[52] Trott O, Olson AJ. AutoDock Vina: Improving the speed and accuracy of docking with a new scoring function, efficient optimization, and multithreading. Journal of Computational Chemistry. 2010;**31**(2):455-461

[53] Kozakov D, Hall DR, Xia B, Porter KA, Padhorny D, Yueh C, et al. The ClusPro web server for protein-protein docking. Nature Protocols. 2017; **12**(2):255

[54] del Alamo D, Sala D, Mchaourab HS, Meiler J. Sampling alternative conformational states of transporters and receptors with AlphaFold2. eLife (2022);**11**:e75751. DOI.org/10.7554/eLife.75751

[55] Pagadala NS, Syed K, Tuszynski J. Software for molecular docking: A review. Biophysical Reviews. 2017; **9**(2):91

[56] Brooijmans N, Kuntz ID. Molecular recognition and docking algorithms. Annual Review of Biophysics and Biomolecular Structure. 2003;**32**:335-373

[57] Sauton N, Lagorce D, Villoutreix BO, Miteva MA. MS-DOCK: Accurate multiple conformation generator and rigid docking protocol for multi-step virtual ligand screening. BMC Bioinformatics. 2008;**9**(1):1-12

[58] DesJarlais RL, Kuntz ID, Sheridan RP, Venkataraghavan R, Dixon JS. Docking flexible ligands to macromolecular receptors by molecular shape. Journal of Medicinal Chemistry. 1986;**29**(11):2149-2153

[59] Rarey M, Kramer B, Lengauer T, Klebe G. A fast flexible docking method using an incremental construction algorithm. Journal of Molecular Biology. 1996;**261**(3):470-489

[60] Lengauer T, Rarey M. Computational methods for biomolecular docking. Current Opinion in Structural Biology. 1996;**6**(3):402-406

[61] Welch WJ, Brown CR. Influence of molecular and chemical chaperones on protein folding. Cell Stress & Chaperones. 1996;**1**(2):109

[62] Halgren TA, Murphy RB, Friesner RA, Beard HS, Frye LL, Pollard WT, Banks JL. Glide: A new approach for rapid, accurate docking and scoring. 2. Enrichment factors in database screening. Journal of Medicinal Chemistry 2004;47(7):1750–1759.

[63] Friesner RA, Banks JL, Murphy RB, Halgren TA, Klicic JJ, Mainz DT, et al. Glide: A new approach for rapid, accurate docking and scoring. 1. Method and assessment of docking accuracy. Journal of Medicinal Chemistry. 2004; **47**(7):1739-1749

[64] Morris GM, Ruth H, Lindstrom W, Sanner MF, Belew RK, Goodsell DS, et al. Software news and updates AutoDock4 and AutoDockTools4: Automated docking with selective receptor

flexibility. Journal of Computational Chemistry. 2009;**30**(16):2785-2791

[65] Dar AM, Mir S. Molecular docking: Approaches, types, applications and basic challenges. J Anal Bioanal Tech. 2017;**8**(2):1-3

[66] Hernández-Santoyo A, Tenorio-Barajas AY, VictorAltuzar V, Vivanco-Cid H, Mendoza-Barrera C. Protein-Protein and Protein-Ligand Docking. In: Ogawa T. editor. Protein Engineering - Technology and Application. London: IntechOpen; 2013. DOI: 10.5772/56376

[67] Cosconati S, Forli S, Perryman AL, Harris R, Goodsell DS, Olson AJ. Virtual screening with AutoDock: Theory and practice. Expert Opinion on Drug Discovery. 2010;**5**(6):597-607

[68] Rizvi SMD, Shakil S, Haneef M. A simple click by click protocol to perform docking: AutoDock 4.2 made easy for non-bioinformaticians. EXCLI Journal. 2013;**12**:831-857

[69] Forli S, Huey R, Pique ME, Sanner MF, Goodsell DS, Olson AJ. Computational protein-ligand docking and virtual drug screening with the AutoDock suite. Nature Protocols. 2016; **11**(5):905-919

[70] Trott O, Olson AJ. AutoDock Vina: Improving the speed and accuracy of docking with a new scoring function, efficient optimization, and multithreading. Journal of Computational Chemistry. 2009;**31**(2):NA-NA

[71] Sandeep G, Nagasree KP, Hanisha M, Kumar MMK. AUDocker LE: A GUI for virtual screening with AUTODOCK Vina. BMC Research Notes. 2011; **4**(1):445

[72] Seeliger D, De Groot BL. Ligand docking and binding site analysis with PyMOL and Autodock/Vina. Journal of Computer-Aided Molecular Design. 2010;**24**(5):417-422

[73] Ravindranath PA, Forli S, Goodsell DS, Olson AJ, Sanner MF. AutoDockFR: Advances in protein-ligand docking with explicitly specified binding site flexibility. PLoS Computational Biology. 2015;**11**(12): e1004586

[74] Hsu KC, Chen YF, Lin SR, Yang JM. Igemdock: A graphical environment of enhancing gemdock using pharmacological interactions and post-screening analysis. BMC Bioinformatics. 2011;**12**(Suppl. 1):S33

[75] Jamkhande PG, Ghante MH, Ajgunde BR. Software based approaches for drug designing and development: A systematic review on commonly used software and its applications. Bull Fac Pharmacy, Cairo Univ. 2017;**55**(2): 203-210

[76] Talluri S. Molecular docking and virtual screening based prediction of drugs for COVID-19. Combinatorial Chemistry & High Throughput Screening. 2021;**24**(5):716-728

[77] Oferkin IV, Katkova EV, Sulimov AV, Kutov DC, Sobolev SI, Voevodin VV, et al. Evaluation of docking target functions by the comprehensive investigation of protein-ligand energy minima. Advances in Bioinformatics. 2015;**2015**:20151-20112

[78] Malmstrom RD, Watowich SJ. Using free energy of binding calculations to improve the accuracy of virtual screening predictions. Journal of Chemical Information and Modeling. 2011;**51**(7):1648-1655

Section 3

Molecular Docking in Drug Repositioning and Virtual Screening

Chapter 5

Development of Nucleic Acid Targeting Molecules: Molecular Docking Approaches and Recent Advances

Mohit Umare, Fai A. Alkathiri and Rupesh Chikhale

Abstract

Molecular docking is a widely used and effective structure-based computational strategy for predicting dynamics between ligands and receptors. Until now the docking software were developed for the protein-ligand interactions and very few docking tools were developed exclusively for the docking of small molecules on the nucleic acid structures like the DNA and RNA. The progress in algorithms and the need for deeper understanding of ligand-nucleic acid interactions more focused, and specialized tools are being developed to explore this hindered area of drug discovery. This chapter is focused on and discus in details about various tools available for docking with nucleic acids and how the rejuvenation of machine learning methods is making its impact on the development of these docking programs.

Keywords: nucleic acids, molecular docking, docking algorithms, machine learning, non-canonical DNA, RNA

1. Introduction

Computer-Aided Drug Design (CADD) has evolved as a cost-effective method of producing potential medications for the treatment of a wide range of diseases [1]. The use of the CADD technique in pharmaceutical research is becoming more common. Recently, there has been a trend in drug design to strategically create effective therapies with multi-targeting effects, better effectiveness, and tolerability, particularly in terms of toxic effects [2, 3]. To assist the exploration, a mix of modern computer approaches, biological research, and synthesizing molecules was developed, and this combinational methodology increased the scope of discoveries [4, 5].

CADD may be generally defined as encompassing both structure- and ligand-based drug design (SBDD and LBDD) [6]. SBDD approaches are based on evidence acquired from an understanding of a target's three-dimensional structure, and they allow rating databases of compounds based on the affinity of ligands to a specific target [7, 8]. LBDD provides a generic technique for understanding links between the structural and compositional features of molecules and their bioactivities. When three-dimensional data for a protein of interest is lacking, this strategy is used [9]. The existing knowledge on molecules and their bioactivity are employed in this approach to produce new possible therapeutic molecules. In this regard, molecular docking is a widely used and effective structure-based computational based strategies for predicting dynamics between ligands and physiological receptors [10, 11].

The molecular docking procedure consists of two main stages: projection of a new molecular configuration including its pose inside the peptide-binding pocket, and evaluation of the pose quality using a scoring function [11, 12]. Around 1975, high-throughput protein isolation, [13] nuclear magnetic resonance spectroscopy, and X-ray crystallography [14] have advanced, primarily leading to improved knowledge of the structural properties of ligand and molecule complex [15].

MD studies, along with many other *in silico* technologies, have grown more frequent and simpler to use in drug development; yet it is not wholly reliant on molecular libraries. Since its inception in the 1980s as among the most mostly utilized procedures, the experimental data collected by MD techniques has developed at an accelerating rate [16]. Nearly annually, programs configured using various methods for MD analysis are produced, considerably boosting pharmaceutical research. The scoring function calculates the binding affinities of produced poses, ranks them, and selects the most advantageous ligand and protein binding modes [17].

The scoring function of an optimum search algorithm should be capable of assessing the physical and chemical characteristics of compounds and the thermodynamics of interactions [18]. The earliest algorithms were created to deal with protein interactions [19]. Over the previous few decades, the progressive development of efficient and comprehensive algorithms with the inclusion of new variables has mirrored computing technical breakthroughs. Kuntz and colleagues at UCSF then utilized a shape pairing method algorithm to keep looking for alternative combinations based on the geometric length between the target and the ligand molecule [20].

The molecular docking technique has risen to prominence in the realm of drug development. Times over the past twenty years, molecular docking has developed as a vital tool for computational drug development, and it has been proved to be more systematic than conventional drug development approaches [16]. The enormous increase in computational capabilities and the rising access of molecule and protein libraries have considerably aided molecular docking. Several docking methodologies have been implemented over the last several years that may be used to dock proteins on peptides with diverse levels of accuracy. Molecular docking was initially intended to be done between a ligand and a target protein, but there is a significant focus on docking between proteins, and nucleic acid-protein-ligand docking, nucleic acid-ligand docking in the recent decade [21].

Methods for addressing the shortcomings of the docking approach are still being researched [22]. Results can be refined, for example, by employing consensus procedures, implementing more stringent scoring techniques to a portion of the filtered library, or employing filters that include interaction fingerprints [23]. Significant effort has also been undertaken to collect inputs from potential binding waters. Identified water molecules as critical for molecule recognition can be considered part of the binding pocket, and prediction can be enhanced by energy contribution by displacing water molecules [24].

2. Methods in molecular docking

2.1 Monte Carlo

In molecular docking studies, the Monte Carlo technique is the use in creation of a randomized conformation of a molecule in a targets active site. The advantage is that this method uses equilibrium statistical method. Rather than attempting to mimic a system's dynamics, it develops states based on the suitable Boltzmann distribution [25]. It determines the initial configuration value. Further, it generates and evaluates a new configuration. Through using Metropolis criteria, it assesses whether the new configuration should be preserved [26]. The Metropolis criteria states that if a new strategy provides better conformation than the previous one, it is recognized immediately. If the combination is not innovative, a probability assessment based on Boltzmann's law is used. If the conclusion passes the likelihood function test, it is approved, and the other arrangement is discarded [27].

2.2 Ligand fit

Ligand fit denotes to a rapid and accurate approach for docking small molecules into targets active sites while considering form as a complementarity. The technique of cavity identification is used in the procedure to discover and produce cavity in the protein as probable binding site locations [28]. For producing ligand poses that are compatible with the receptor binding site shape, a shape similarity screening is paired along with a Monte Carlo parametric analysis. A grid-based technique for analyzing energies between protein and ligand is used to reduce candidate poses with respect to the active site. A non-linear interpolation approach drastically reduces errors caused by grid interpolation [27, 28].

2.3 Point complimentary

Here on grounds of the complementarity of the interatomic contacts, a technique for docking a drug into a binding pocket in an enzyme is disclosed. Docking is accomplished by increasing a complementarity function that is reliant on the atomic surface area of contact as well as the elemental composition of the interacting atoms [29]. Although the target and ligand molecules are viewed as inflexible entities, mobility of a restricted range of residues bordering the binding site can also be considered. These techniques of molecular docking are focused on comparing the shapes and/or chemical properties of different molecules [26].

2.4 Fragment based

Fragment-based drug discovery (FBDD) is a novel strategy that is increasingly being used to improve hit recognition for previously thought intractable biological targets. FBDD, in specifically, uncovers small ligands (300 Da) capable of binding to pharmacologically important macromolecules with micromolar affinity [30].

2.5 Distance geometry

Even though it is primarily known as a tool for predicting the solution conformation of compounds from NMR data, distance geometry is a basic and effective tool for generating approximation models of complicated chemical formations [31]. Distance geometry is a basic geometrical approach that builds structures directly to fulfill model requirements; this does not involve an initial conformational or force field variables. The approach simply handles flexible rings without any extra attention or adjustment. Distance geometry is also distinct in that it works well together with qualitative data: a significant number of estimated distance boundaries are more useful in creating a model than a limited handful of highly exact distances [12, 31].

3. Nucleic acid docking

Nucleic acids (NAs) are biological macromolecules which can be broken down into phosphoric acid, sugars, and mixture of organic bases like purines and pyrimidines [32]. These can occur in various forms and constitute the building blocks like the DNA and RNA. These are essential for various cellular process including cell division and protein synthesis [33, 34]. Due to their crucial role in cell division, DNA, RNA, and their alternate structures have become target of choice for drug discovery in case of cancer drug discovery, infectious diseases, and rare diseases [35–38]. The NA modulators act by interfering with DNA replication process which affect the cell proliferation, transcription and ultimately inhibition of gene expression [39]. These agents can modulate the functioning of the RNA resulting in altered transcription and translation processes [40]. These modulators could be small molecule ligands, peptide or macromolecules, these can interact with the NAs by various mechanisms like intercalation, molecular cross-linking, DNA or RNA strand cleavage, and interference at the site of NA-protein interactions (**Figure 1**) [40, 41].

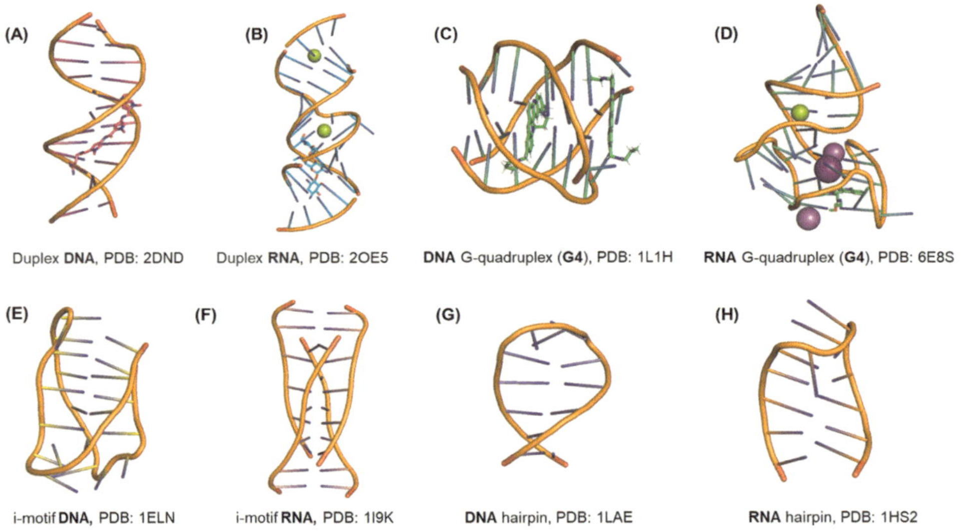

Figure 1.
The commonly known NA structures with and without bound ligands; (A) duplex DNA structure with a bound antitumour drug, distamycin, PDB: 2DND [42]; (B) duplex RNA structure with a bound aminoglycoside antibiotic, apramycin, PDB: 2OE5 [43]; (C) DNA G-quadruplex in complex with the di-substituted amino alkylamido acridine compound (G4), PDB: 1L1H [44]; (D) RNA G-quadruplex (G4) crystal structures of TO1-biotin complexes of mango-III, a structure-guided mutant mango-III (A10U), PDB: 6E8S [45]; (E) i-motif DNA, a fragment of the vertebrate telomere which folds intramolecularly, PDB: 1ELN [46]; (F) i-motif RNA, a oligodeoxynucleotides with stretches of cytidine residues associate into a four-stranded structure, PDB: 1I9K [47]; (G) DNA hairpin, solution structure of the PdG-containing hairpin PDB: 1LAE [48]; (H) RNA hairpin, solution structure of RNA hairpin loop, PDB: 1HS2 [49].

Recent advancement in crystallization techniques, oligonucleotide synthesis, methods for structure determination like the NMR, crystal diffraction and cryo-EM has allowed for enrichment of structural data for NAs [50, 51]. The protein data bank (PDB) is an open source repository where these structures are deposited and curated [52]. There are more than 730 DNA-ligand and 523 RNA-ligand co-crystallized structures in the PDB and these would keep increasing [53]. Structural data of NAs helps in the investigation of the possible binding of ligands into the target, a co-crystallized structure provides with a bound ligand which helps understand the binding or active site in the given NAs. These co-crystallized molecules offer an excellent opportunity to perform structure-based and ligand-based drug discovery experiments and apply various other computational methods for drug discovery of NAs therapeutics. The most widely used method in computational drug design is molecular docking studies. The algorithms available for performing molecular docking are basically made for ligand-protein docking. There are several similarities like the protein and NAs follow similar physicochemical binding principles. However, these algorithms often fail to lack of sufficient sampling of the conformation space in case of NA docking to reasons of non-specific scoring functions [54]. Most of the target protein molecules contain a hydrophobic binding site whereas, the NAs consist of a rather more solvent-exposed binding pocket with higher polarity and charge density [55]. These are the major differences between the proteins and NAs as targets in molecular docking. Most of these algorithms are focused on the protein target molecules and need to consider parameters that need to be included in the program for NAs docking. NAs particularly the RNAs are very flexible owing to their charge, intrinsic atomic arrangements, and movements due to the presence of ligands. This flexibility is not considered by most of the programs as they consider NAs as rigid bodies [56]. Some programs like MORDOR are available that allows for the flexibility of the NAs and the ligands [57]. It applies molecular mechanics minimisation restraints based on the data from the X-ray and NMR experimental data [58]. There are several shortfalls to these methods, they are marred by slow speed, minimisation stages are slow, and time consuming, and large library screening is not feasible. Other NA specific methods reported were ensemble docking based on structural information from the X-ray structures or NMR or structures from the normal-mode analysis of an MD simulation [59–61]. The presence of water molecules and metal ions add to the complications in NAs docking. The water molecules and metal ions are essential for the stability and functioning of the NAs, this makes their presence in any docking protocol imperative. The metal ions in case of NAs like the i-Motif and G-quadruplex are necessary for the formation and stability of the structure [62, 63]. Various algorithms that considers these challenges in NAs docking are discussed in the section scoring function.

4. Recent developments in docking tools for nucleic acid

There are several types of small molecules that interact with the NAs and its alternate forms. These can be subdivided into double stranded DNA/RNA (ds-DNA and ds-RNA) binding, G-quadruplex DNA/RNA (G4-DNA and G4-RNA) binding, i-Motif DNA/RNA (iM-DNA and iM-RNA) binding ligands and ligands interacting with other DNA structures like hairpins [62, 63]. These ligands can also be classified based on their mechanism of binding to the DNA, for example covalent binding and intercalators. Several review articles have discussed these ligands in more details in the past [64]. The lab-based experiments and further crystallization experiments are costly and time consuming and hence to assist with these efforts molecular modeling and docking tools are used widely to find the most suitable ligand. Most of the available molecular docking tools have been developed for protein-ligand docking. These tools have been used for NA-ligand docking irrespective of the fact that these tools do not consider the NAs as flexible moieties and thus do not consider the most important feature of NAs. The other type of docking interaction that NA undergo is with the proteins, Protein-NAs docking [65]. There are several algorithms that are used to perform NA-protein docking as mentioned in the table number 1. Earlier reports in NA-ligand docking dealt with finding correct docking conformations based on RMSD to the native co-crystallized ligand. Autodock and Surflex were used to dock several ligands like pentamidine, daunorubicin, distamycin and ellipticine in the minor groove of the ds-DNA. It was observed that Surflex performed better over Autodock in speed of operation and results with lower reference RMSD [66]. Several algorithms have been published and are available for NAs-ligand docking like, GRAMM, FTDock, 3D-DOCK, HEX, Dot and DoT2, HADDOCK, PatchDock, SymmDock, ParaDock, GOLD, Glide [67], NPDcok and HDOCK (**Table 1**). The most recent NA-ligand docking tools are NLDock, LigandRNA and DOCK 6.

The DOCK algorithm developed by the Kuntz lab has been traditionally a protein-ligand docking program. However, the most recent development of the series is

Algorithms	Acronym	Principle	Reference
Geometric Recognition Algorithm to identify Molecular surface complementarity.	GRAMM	Rigid docking uses fast Fourier transformation, shape-based complementarity.	[68]
Fourier Transform rigid-body Docking	FTDock	Use and implementation of the biochemical and electrostatic information of the DNA and host protein or DNA.	[69]
Initial grid-based shape complementarity search	3D-Dock	Featured backbone refinement, side chain optimization and energy calculations.	[70]
Spherical polar Fourier correlations	HEX	Docking pairs of proteins by using spherical polar Fourier correlations to accelerate the search for candidate low-energy conformations.	[71]
Rapid computation of the electrostatic potential energy between two proteins or other charged molecules.	Dot and Dot2 (Daughter of Turnip)	Automated construction of improved biophysical models based on molecular coordinates, provides for flexibility with grid size and allows improved rescoring method. Uses Poisson-Boltzmann methods.	[72]
High Ambiguity Driven protein-protein Docking	HADDOCK	Uses Ambiguous Interaction Restraints (AIRs), takes up information form the biophysical, biochemical interactions found in the NMR or crystal structure.	[73]
Geometry-based molecular docking algorithm	PatchDock	Aims at finding good molecular shape complementarity.	[74]
Geometry-based docking algorithm for the prediction of a cyclically symmetric complex	SymmDock	It aims to find symmetric cyclic transformations.	[75]

Algorithms	Acronym	Principle	Reference
ab initio protein–DNA docking algorithm	ParaDock	Geometric complementarity-based docking.	[76]
Protein-Nucleic acid docking	NPDock	It predicts the protein–nucleic acid structures interactions by clustering the best-scored models and ranking the refined solutions.	[77]
Hybrid docking	HDOCK	Template based modeling and free docking.	[78]
Genetic Optimisation for Ligand Docking	Gold	Explores full range of ligand conformational flexibility, loosely bound water molecules in the binding site or the active site.	[79]
RNA – ligand interactions	$DrugScore^{RNA}$	Uses experimental structures as reference and applies distance-dependent pair potentials with reference.	[80]
Molecular Recognition with a Driven dynamics Optimize R	MORDOR	Explores the electrostatic, van der Waals forces. Takes consideration of dihedral angle, torsion angle, and bond lengths. CHARMM or AMBER based scoring functions and uses implicit solvent models.	[61]
Binding mode predictions	AutoDock AutoDock Vina	Uses simulated annealing method for docking, flexible ligand and some extent of receptor flexibility.	[81–84]
Fully automated flexible docking	Surflex	Uses surface-based molecular similarity method to generate suitable poses for molecular fragments.	[85]
RiboDock	rDock	It uses stochastic and deterministic search techniques and generates low energy ligand poses.	[86]
Nucleic acid-Protein Docking	NPDock	Makes use of clustering of best score models.	[77]
Nucleic acid-Ligand Docking	NLDock	ITScore-NL scoring function used, it makes the use of stacking and electrostatic potentials.	[87, 88]
RNA-Ligand docking	LigandRNA	Makes use of grid-based algorithm and potentials derived from experimentally solved RNA-ligand complexes.	[89]
Iterative knowledge-based scoring function for nucleic acid–ligand interactions	ITScore-NL	Physics based iterative methods used. Makes use of atomic and distance dependent pair potentials. Uses stacking interactions and electrostatic effects.	[88]
Ranking-based sampling algorithm	DOCK 6	Dominant electrostatics and charges from waters were considered.	[90]

Table 1.
List of NA-ligand docking tools with their names and principle of working and algorithms.

DOCK6 which has the special feature to dock small molecules on the NAs. DOCK6 have significant progress in ligand orientation and conformational sampling which has led to significant improvement in the accuracy of docking for the large and flexible molecules over the NAs. It uses a sampling algorithm 'anchor-and-grow' which allows a cluster-based pruning with controlled cut-off of 25 kcal/mol. This flexibility in the upper limit allows for ranked orientation and improves prediction near the binding site. DOCK 6 uses the MD parameters like the AMBER GB/SA and PB/SA for predicting and ranking the poses and the effect of presence of metal ions and the water molecules in the binding site. The NLDock developed by the Huang lab uses ITScoreNL which is an iterative knowledge-based scoring function. The ITScoreNL uses a statistical mechanics based interactive algorithm. It uses the information from a training set of experimentally determined structures in the protein data bank (PDB). This scoring function consist of atomic, distance dependent pair potential, stacking interaction, and electrostatic effects. Results from ITScoreNL significantly improve the performance in binding and affinity prediction for the NAs-ligand complex. Recent advances and enrichment of the RNA structures in the PDB let to the development of LigandRNA. It uses the 3D information from the available RNA structures. A potential is obtained using the inverse Boltzmann scheme which considers the ligand poses that are favorable and exhibit interactions fitting the maxima of the statistical distribution of RNA-ligand atom contacts derived from the RNA-ligand co-crystal structures. This method is dedicated to scoring and ranking ligand poses in their RNA three-dimensional structure with correct intramolecular interactions while maintaining high accuracy and precision. These recent tools have given larger momentum to screening of ligands for NAs with better accuracy and speed.

5. Scoring functions

Molecular docking is quickly becoming a valuable technique in drug development and molecular modeling fields. The precision of the selected scoring function, that can lead and identify ligand positions when hundreds of potential ligand positions are created, determines the effectiveness of molecular docking [11, 91, 92]. The scoring function can also be used to forecast binding affinity and discover possible drug candidates for a specific protein of interest, as well as to define the binding mode and location of a molecule [93]. In lead optimization, scoring functions serve three main purposes: first, they recognize the best location of a ligand's binding to a protein based on the scoring function; second, they estimate the absolute binding affinity between the protein and ligand; and third, they perform virtual screening, which can identify possible drug leads for a given target protein by finding a sizable molecule database [93].

The most recent scoring functions for protein-ligand interactions using a new categorization that divides the scoring functions into force-field-based, empirical, and knowledge-based SFs. Ongoing study has drastically enhanced the research for scoring functions, particularly in protein-ligand interactions.

5.1 Physics-based scoring functions

Direct computation of the associations between both the atoms of a protein and a ligand is possible using physics-based SFs. Owing to the consideration of solvation, enthalpy, and entropy, physics-based SFs are suited to calculate binding free energy among proteins and ligands with significantly improved prediction performance than other forms of SFs [94]. These are founded on solvation models, force fields, and quantum mechanics techniques. The van der Waals and electrostatic interactions between the protein and ligand atom pairs are added up in the conventional force field-based SF, which considers the energy-contributing role of enthalpy, to estimate the binding energy [95].

Pairwise atomic interactions between the ligand and protein are the focus of the fundamental equation in the classical method. R is the distance between atomic centres, q is the fractional charge on every atom, and e is the dielectric constant. The A and B parameters are determined for every pair of various atom type combinations [96].

$$\Delta G_{bind} = \sum_{i=1}^{ligand} \sum_{j=1}^{protein} \left[\frac{A_{ij}}{R_{ij}^{12}} - \frac{B_{ij}}{R_{ij}^{6}} + \frac{q_i q_j}{\varepsilon R_{ij}} \right]$$

5.2 Empirical scoring functions

Empirical SFs calculate a complex's binding energy by adding up the essential energy components for binding affinity, such as hydrophobic effects, hydrogen bonds, steric conflicts, and so on. There are two study paths in empirical SFs. One approach is to use a usually high labeled training data to optimize protein complexes; the other is to pick appropriate energy terms using progressive parameters and methodical selection of the target molecule [92, 97].

5.3 Knowledge-based scoring functions

Predicated on the reverse Boltzmann statistic concept, knowledge-based SFs compute the appropriate pairwise potential in terms of 3D structures of a wide range of complexes. The rate of distinct atom pairs at different distances is thought to be connected to the interactions between two atoms, which translates the rate through the distance-dependent potential of mean force [18]. When tried to compare to physics and empirical SFs, knowledge-based SFs have the largest benefit in terms of processing cost and prediction accuracy. Unfortunately, knowledge-based SFs have a tough time locating the reference state [98].

5.4 DrugScoreRNA

Interactions of protein with protein, DNA, and ligand have all been studied using knowledge-based techniques. DrugScoreRNA is the first knowledge-based technique to scoring RNA-ligand complexes. Because of the small percentage of experimental measurements of RNA-ligand combinations, it was thought that obtaining statistically meaningful potentials was improbable [80].

The fact that the binding (free) energy landscape derived by such prospects is more focused than in the context of all other knowledge-based SFs or AutoDock may be taken into consideration as one of the factors contributing to DrugScoreRNA's effectiveness in docking [18]. This is anticipated to result in a quicker docking converging to a global solution, or, put another way, a lower probability that the configurational search would get stale in a local minimum. Reasonable correlation exists between experimental binding free energies and binding scores estimated by DrugScoreRNA [99].

5.5 RiboDock

The growing understanding of the significance of RNA in fundamental biological processes has lately made them more appealing as prospective therapeutic targets. To find small compounds that may selectively bind to identified locations in RNA molecules and inhibit or otherwise modify their function, a greater number of scientifically confirmed RNA three- dimensional structures were available. This allowed for structure-based searches for these molecules [100]. The access to high resolution structures of RNA-ligand complexes substantially facilitates the investigation of the atomic intricacies of RNA-ligand contacts. Furthermore, it is difficult to determine the physical structure of RNA and its interactions, and it is now unable to do so in a high-throughput way. This is what inspired the creation of source code for simulating the configurations of RNA-ligand complexes based on the known structures of RNA targets. Many of these advancements were motivated by comparable strategies used earlier for protein-ligand complex modeling [89, 100].

One of the first to develop a scoring function specifically for RNA-ligand complexes was done in 2004 by Morley and Afshar. They added the empirical regression-based tool RiboDock (or rDock) to their own high-throughput docking tool to handle RNA-ligand structures [101]. This technique was, unfortunately, parameterized and tested on a small sample size of just 10 RNA molecules. Ligand intramolecular, intermolecular, site intramolecular, and external constraint factors are weighted together to form the rDock master score function. The major terminology of importance is S^{intra}, which stands for the RNA-ligand interaction score. According on the provided ligand configuration, S^{intra} provides the ligand's energy transfer. Similar to S^{site}, this term denotes the comparative energy of the active site's variable regions [100, 101].

5.6 LigandRNA

As discussed in the above section, the importance of RNA in fundamental biological processes has grown the scientific community interest in the research area of Nucleic Acid-Ligand docking. Another Scoring function developed for the similar function was LigandRNA [89].

The RNA-ligand complexes were computationally solved using the LigandRNA approach, which uses a grid-based algorithm and a knowledge-based SFs obtained from ligand-binding domains. LigandRNA requires two files as inputs: an RNA receptor file and a ligand poses file. It produces a list of poses ranked by their score as an output [100]. The potential is calculated using the inverse Boltzmann method, which assumes that only ligand poses with interactions that meet the maximum of the statistical distribution of RNA-ligand atom contacts generated from empirically established structures of RNA-ligand complexes are advantageous. Thus, according to their value, the supplied ligand poses are sorted, and this score would be used to assess the relative effectiveness of binding [89].

5.7 MM/PBSA and MM/GBSA

The molecular mechanics energies combined with the Poisson–Boltzmann or generalized Born and surface area continuum solvation (MM/PBSA and MM/GBSA) are the popular techniques for estimating the free energy of the binding of ligand molecules to the target protein. In MM/PBSA, the free energy of a state, that is, P, L or PL in the following equation, is estimated from the following sum [102].

$G = E_{bnd} + E_{el} + E_{vdW} + G_{pol} + G_{np} - TS.$

$E_{bnd:}$ Bonded (bond, angle and dihedral) energy.

E_{el}: Electrostatic Energy.

E_{vdW}: van der Waals interactions.

G_{pol}: polar contribution to the solvation free energy.

G_{np}: non-polar contribution to the solvation free energy.

To calculate the MM/GBSA free energy, the system of relevance is first modeled either using Metropolis Monte Carlo or molecular dynamics (MD), with pose is being obtained at set intervals and for each pose the free energy is calculated by the above equation. The continuum-solvation technique, the dielectric constant, the charges, the sample selection, and the entropies have a significant impact on the outcomes. The approaches frequently exaggerate the differences between different ligand groups [103]. In actual use, it frequently produces outcomes of middling quality, frequently outperforming docking, and scoring. However, because of the findings' substantial reliance on the continuum solvation used, either the absolute affinities or the methodology is invalid [103, 104].

5.8 Molecular recognition with a driven dynamics optimizer (MORDOR)

The fixed nature of the protein target is drawback in most of the docking tools. To overcome this and to explore the dynamic nature of the target Molecular Recognition with a Driven dynamics Optimizer (MORDOR) tool was developed. MORDOR allows induced-fit type of docking algorithm. A new RNA stabilizing loop can be formed by the ligand, which could move bases [105].

MORDOR uses a unique conformational field search technique to achieve this goal, enabling a productive thorough search while docking. Utilizing a driving force to move the ligand, this method combines molecular minimization technique. By applying an extra RMSD kind of force, the ligand explores the receptor surface after beginning from any pose in and around the receptor. It is crucial to research induced fit with MORDOR when docking proteins, especially RNA. Drugs do not often bind a conventional form of nucleic acid, according to the architectures of nucleic acid-drug complexes. Also, more control over the docking process is provided by the allowance of an infinite number of restraints. Contrarily, it seems from known drug-nucleic acid binding structures that the small molecule ligands frequently replace bases, leading to a local restructuring of the nucleic acid. A drug development process will have a far better chance of being successful if flexible docking for RNA is used [61, 105].

5.9 Dock-RNA

Numerous biological activities, including the production and control of gene activity, depend on nucleic acid-ligand interactions. As a result, nucleic acid molecules like RNAs have grown in importance as pharmacological targets and knowing the structural characteristics of RNA-ligand complexes is essential to deriving treatment strategies. The nucleic acid-ligand docking method is divided into two stages: The model chooses a preliminary set of potential poses during the first stage using a different computer algorithm for the Born radiuses in the electrical charges; with in second stage, a stringent scoring function is utilized to arrange the poses to identify the top molecules [106].

The scoring function of the molecular docking program is dependent on the shift in free energy caused by RNA-ligand binding. It aggregates comparable ligand poses into clusters based on geometrical similarity and ranks the grouped poses based on the binding affinity. Because it separates itself from other models by sampling all potential interaction site and poses globally, the findings above highlight the relevance poses. Unfortunately, the RLDOCK approach is difficult to apply to big target and ligand sets. The time-consuming selection of the complex formation produces prohibitively small processing effectiveness of the approach in complexes with a big RNA such as ribosomal RNA or ligands with the more than 12 rotatable bonds [107, 108].

6. Role of machine learning and artificial intelligence

Machine learning (ML) specially the Deep learning methods (DL) and Artificial intelligence (AI) has rapidly developed and is being used in drug discovery. ML in drug discovery is used to improve the existing scoring functions or to develop a new scoring function for virtual screening studies. The existing scoring functions can be improved by refining their empirical function's weights. Most of the ML based scoring function improvements has been seen in the protein-ligand docking and their virtual screening domain. The ML methods being used are Random Forest methods [109], Gradient boosting trees method [110], Support vector machine methods [111], Multi-layer perceptron methods [112], Convolutional neural network methods [113], and Graph neural network [114]. The scoring functions for NAs-ligand interactions can be classified into force-field based, empirical, knowledge-based and machine learning based. The machine learning based scoring functions can capture intrinsic nonlinearities in the training set without imposing a predetermined functional form. The most important feature that separates the ML methods from others is that ML maps the ligands to a potential energy landscape, it is inherently flexible, and the mapping relationship works without the addition of extensive physicochemical knowledge. However, the use of ML in NAs binding ligands discovery comes with certain challenges as well. First, the mapping relationships generated by ML are not always interpretable and the second, ML models for NAs could find difficult to make accurate predictions for complexes out of the training sets.

For the NA-ligand complex interactions two ML based scoring functions were recently developed, RNAPoser [115] and AnnapuRNA [116]. The RNAPoser uses a set of 80 RNA-ligand experimental structures as dataset and investigates the 'nativeness' of the RNA-ligands poses. This program uses machine learning methods to train a set of pose classifiers that would estimate the position of the ligands in the experimental structures. These poses are defined as fingerprints which are encoded as local RNA environment surrounding the ligand. This method uses the leave-one-out training and testing approach where about 80% of the native poses were recovered within 2.5 Å. The classification is done based on ranking of ligands and scoring from machine learning classifiers, which were able to recover the native like poses. The validation set for the method returned recovery of native poses for more than 60% of the cases. These were found to be better than the poses with higher docking scores. Another recent development in the NA-ligand docking improvement is AnnapuRNA. It is a machine learning-based statistical scoring function which can evaluate the quality of RNA-Ligand complex structure predicted by a computational docking program and thus help in validation of the docking results. It uses the information like the initial ligand conformation, the docking program and the scoring function used by the docking program. The training set is derived from the experimental data available on the PDB and it uses the *k*NN (*k*-Nearest Neighbors) and Deep Learning (multi-layer feedforward artificial neural network) as ML algorithms. This program supports a various docking program like the AutoDock, AutoDock Vina, Dock6, rDock, iDock, LigandRNA, and several other NAs specific programs.

7. Conclusion

In this chapter we have overviewed various important aspects in development of small molecule inhibitors for NAs and various docking software specific and non-specific for NAs-ligand docking. We have also reviewed various docking programs, algorithms and scoring functions, their advantages and lacune and challenges in the discovery of novel NAs binding ligands. Until recently most of the algorithms were focused on protein-ligand docking but now slowly programs specific for NAs are appearing in the molecular docking space. The progress in ML and AI has led to an advantage for development of NA specific algorithms. However, there is lot of scope for development of NA-docking specific programs, structural variations of NA also pose a challenge for the new programs. However, it is possible to convert these challenges into opportunities as the need for better NA targeting ligands are high in demand specifically due to the resurgence of viral infections and other infectious disease.

Acknowledgements

FA acknowledges the support provided by Department of Pharmaceutics, College of Pharmacy, King Saud University, Riyadh, Saudi Arabia.

Author details

Mohit Umare[1], Fai A. Alkathiri[2] and Rupesh Chikhale[3*]

1 Tata Consultancy Services Limited, Pune, India

2 Department of Pharmaceutics, College of Pharmacy, King Saud University, Riyadh, Saudi Arabia

3 UCL School of Pharmacy, London, UK

*Address all correspondence to: rupeshchikhale7@gmail.com

References

[1] Tang Y, Zhu W, Chen K, Jiang H. New technologies in computer-aided drug design: Toward target identification and new chemical entity discovery. Drug Discovery Today: Technologies. 2006;**3**: 307-313

[2] Kiriiri GK, Njogu PM, Mwangi AN. Exploring different approaches to improve the success of drug discovery and development projects: A review. Future Journal of Pharmaceutical Sciences. 2020;**6**(1):27

[3] Yu W, MacKerell AD Jr. Computer-aided drug design methods. Methods in Molecular Biology. 2017;**1520**:85-106

[4] Nicolaou KC. Organic synthesis: The art and science of replicating the molecules of living nature and creating others like them in the laboratory. Proceedings of the Royal Society A: Mathematical, Physical and Engineering Sciences. 2014;**470**(2163):20130690

[5] Atanasov AG, Zotchev SB, Dirsch VM, Orhan IE, Banach M, Rollinger JM, et al. Natural products in drug discovery: Advances and opportunities. Nature Reviews Drug Discovery. 2021;**20**(3):200-216

[6] Aparoy P, Reddy KK, Reddanna P. Structure, and ligand-based drug design strategies in the development of novel 5-LOX inhibitors. Current Medicinal Chemistry. 2012;**19**(22):3763-3778

[7] Meng XY, Zhang HX, Mezei M, Cui M. Molecular docking: A powerful approach for structure-based drug discovery. Current Computer-Aided Drug Design. 2011;7(2):146-157

[8] Yasuo N, Sekijima M. Improved method of structure-based virtual screening via interaction-energy-based learning. Journal of Chemical Information and Modeling. 2019;**59**(3): 1050-1061

[9] Bacilieri M, Moro S. Ligand-based drug design methodologies in drug discovery process: An overview. Current Drug Discovery Technologies. 2006;**3**: 155-165

[10] Sivakumar KC, Haixiao J, Naman CB, Sajeevan TP. Prospects of multitarget drug designing strategies by linking molecular docking and molecular dynamics to explore the protein–ligand recognition process. Drug Development Research. 2020;**81**(6):685-699

[11] Silakari O, Singh PK. Chapter 6 - Molecular docking analysis: Basic technique to predict drug-receptor interactions. In: Silakari O, Singh PKBTC and EP of M and I in DD, editors. Concepts and Experimental Protocols of Modelling and Informatics in Drug Design. Academic Press; 2021. pp. 131-155

[12] Guedes IA, de Magalhães CS, Dardenne LE. Receptor-ligand molecular docking. Biophysical Reviews. 2013/12/ 21. 2014;**6**(1):75-87

[13] Koehn J, Hunt I. High-throughput protein production (HTPP): A review of enabling technologies to expedite protein production. Methods in Molecular Biology. 2009;**498**:1-18

[14] Jhoti H, Cleasby A, Verdonk M, Williams G. Fragment-based screening using X-ray crystallography and NMR spectroscopy. Current Opinion in Chemical Biology. 2007;**11**(5):485-493

[15] Kim Y, Bigelow L, Borovilos M, Dementieva I, Duggan E,

Eschenfeldt W, et al. Chapter 3. High-throughput protein purification for x-ray crystallography and NMR. Advances in Protein Chemistry and Structural Biology. 2008;**75**:85-105

[16] Pinzi L, Rastelli G. Molecular docking: Shifting paradigms in drug discovery. International Journal of Molecular Sciences. 2019;**20**(18):4331

[17] Stanzione F, Giangreco I, Cole JC. Use of molecular docking computational tools in drug discovery. Progress in Medicinal Chemistry. 1st ed. Vol. 60. Elsevier B.V.; 2021. pp. 273-343

[18] Ferrara P, Gohlke H, Price DJ, Klebe G, Brooks CL 3rd. Assessing scoring functions for protein-ligand interactions. Journal of Medicinal Chemistry. 2004;**47**(12):3032-3047

[19] Hoskins J, Lovell S, Blundell TL. An algorithm for predicting protein-protein interaction sites: Abnormally exposed amino acid residues and secondary structure elements. Protein Science. 2006;**15**(5):1017-1029

[20] DesJarlais RL, Sheridan RP, Seibel GL, Dixon JS, Kuntz ID, Venkataraghavan R. Using shape complementarity as an initial screen in designing ligands for a receptor binding site of known three-dimensional structure. Journal of Medicinal Chemistry. 1988 Apr;**31**(4):722-729

[21] Torres PHM, Sodero ACR, Jofily P, Silva-Jr FP. Key topics in molecular docking for drug design. International Journal of Molecular Sciences. 2019;**20**(18):4574

[22] Yuriev E, Ramsland PA. Latest developments in molecular docking: 2010–2011 in review. Journal of Molecular Recognition. 2013;**26**(5):215-239

[23] Lionta E, Spyrou G, Vassilatis DK, Cournia Z. Structure-based virtual screening for drug discovery: Principles, applications and recent advances. Current Topics in Medicinal Chemistry. 2014;**14**(16):1923-1938

[24] Maurer M, Oostenbrink C. Water in protein hydration and ligand recognition. Journal of Molecular Recognition. 2019;**32**(12):e2810 e2810

[25] Zivkovic M, Zlatanovic M, Zlatanovic N, Golubović M, Veselinović AM. The application of the combination of Monte Carlo optimization method based QSAR modeling and molecular docking in drug design and development. Mini Reviews in Medicinal Chemistry. 2020;**20**(14):1389-1402

[26] Zivkovic M, Zlatanovic M, Zlatanovic N, Golubović M, Veselinović AM. The Application of the Combination of Monte Carlo Optimization Method based QSAR. Modeling and Molecular Docking in Drug Design and Development. Mini Rev Med Chem. 2020;**20**(14):1389-402

[27] Salmaso V, Moro S. Bridging molecular docking to molecular dynamics in exploring ligand-protein recognition process: An overview. Frontiers in Pharmacology. 2018;**9**. Available online From: https://www.frontiersin.org/articles/10.3389/fphar.2018.00923. DOI=10.3389/fphar.2018.00923. ISSN=1663-9812

[28] Venkatachalam C, Jiang X, Oldfield T, Waldman M. LigandFit: A novel method for the shape-directed rapid docking of ligands to protein active sites. Journal of Molecular Graphics & Modelling. 2003;**21**:289-307

[29] Sobolev V, Wade RC, Vriend G, Edelman M. Molecular docking using

surface complementarity. Proteins. 1996; **25**(1):120-129

[30] Murray CW, Rees DC. The rise of fragment-based drug discovery. Nature Chemistry. 2009;**1**(3):187-192

[31] Blaney JM, Dixon JS. Distance geometry in molecular modeling. In: Drug Discov Design. 1994. pp. 299-335. DOI: 10.1002/9780470125823.ch6. ISSN: 9780471188667

[32] Yamada Y. Nucleic acid drugs—Current status, issues, and expectations for exosomes. Cancers (Basel). 2021;**13**(19):5002. DOI: 10.3390/cancers13195002. PMID: 34638486; PMCID: PMC8508492

[33] The Structure of Nucleic Acids and Their Role in Protein Synthesis - PMC [Internet]. [cited 2022 Jul 7]. Available from: https://www.ncbi.nlm.nih.gov/pmc/articles/PMC2603672/

[34] Carrey EA, Perrett D. Nucleic acids, purine, and pyrimidine nucleotides and nucleosides: Physiology, toxicology, and dietary sources. Encyclopedia of Human Nutrition. 2013;**3–4**:189-196

[35] Kiwerska K, Szyfter K. DNA repair in cancer initiation, progression, and therapy—A double-edged sword. Journal of Applied Genetics. 2019;**60**(3):329. [Internet] [cited 2022 Jul 7]. Available from: /pmc/articles/PMC6803590/

[36] Alhmoud JF, Woolley JF, al Moustafa AE, Malki MI. DNA damage/repair Management in Cancers. Cancers (Basel). 2020;**12**(4):1050. DOI: 10.3390/cancers12041050. PMID: 32340362; PMCID: PMC7226105

[37] Lee JH, Xiong F, Li W. Enhancer RNAs in cancer: Regulation, mechanisms and therapeutic potential. RNA Biology. 2020;**17**(11):1550-1559 [Internet] [cited 2022 Jul 7]. Available from: https://pubmed.ncbi.nlm.nih.gov/31916476/

[38] Knoch J, Kamenisch Y, Kubisch C, Berneburg M. Rare hereditary diseases with defects in DNA-repair. European Journal of Dermatology. 2012;**22**(4): 443-455 [Internet]. [cited 2022 Jul 7]. Available from: https://pubmed.ncbi.nlm.nih.gov/22436139/

[39] Babur Ö, Demir E, Gönen M, Sander C, Dogrusoz U. Discovering modulators of gene expression. Nucleic Acids Research. 2010;**38**(17):5648-5656 [Internet]. [cited 2022 Jul 7]. Available from: https://academic.oup.com/nar/article/38/17/5648/1029365

[40] Zamani F, Suzuki T. Synthetic RNA modulators in drug discovery. Journal of Medicinal Chemistry. 2021;**64**(11): 7110-7155 [Internet]. [cited 2022 Jul 7]. Available from: https://pubs.acs.org/doi/abs/10.1021/acs.jmedchem.1c00154

[41] Bhagavan NV, Ha CE. Structure and Properties of DNA, In: Bhagavan NV, Ha CE. editors. Essentials of Medical Biochemistry. Academic Press. 2011. pp. 275-286. Available from: https://www.sciencedirect.com/science/article/pii/B9780120954612000217. DOI: 10.1016/B978-0-12-095461-2.00021-7. ISBN 9780120954612

[42] Coll M, Frederick CA, Wang AH, Rich A. A bifurcated hydrogen-bonded conformation in the d(a.T) base pairs of the DNA dodecamer d (CGCAAATTTGCG) and its complex with distamycin. Proceedings of the National Academy of Sciences of the United States of America. 1987;**84**(23): 8385-8389 [Internet]. [cited 2022 Jul 8]. Available from: https://www.pnas.org

[43] Hermann T, Tereshko V, Skripkin E, Patel DJ. Apramycin recognition by the

human ribosomal decoding site. Blood Cells, Molecules, and Diseases. 2007; **38**(3):193-198

[44] Haider SM, Parkinson GN, Neidle S. Structure of a G-quadruplex–ligand complex. Journal of Molecular Biology. 2003;**326**(1):117-125

[45] Trachman RJ, Autour A, Jeng SCY, Abdolahzadeh A, Andreoni A, Cojocaru R, et al. Structure and functional reselection of the mango-III fluorogenic RNA aptamer. Nature Chemical Biology. 2019;**15**(5):472-479 [Internet]. [cited 2022 Jul 8]. Available from: https://www.nature.com/articles/s41589-019-0267-9

[46] Phan AT, Guéron M, Leroy JL. The solution structure and internal motions of a fragment of the cytidine-rich strand of the human telomere. Journal of Molecular Biology. 2000;**299**(1):123-144

[47] Snoussi K, Nonin-Lecomte S, Leroy JL. The RNA i-motif. Journal of Molecular Biology. 2001;**309**(1):139-153

[48] Weisenseel JP, Reddy GR, Marnett LJ, Stone MP. Structure of the 1, N2-propanodeoxyguanosine adduct in a three-base DNA hairpin loop derived from a palindrome in the salmonella typhimurium hisD3052 gene. Chemical Research in Toxicology. 2002;**15**(2): 140-152 [Internet]. [cited 2022 Jul 8]. Available from: https://pubs.acs.org/doi/abs/10.1021/tx010107f

[49] Zhang H, Fountain MA, Krugh TR. Structural characterization of a six-nucleotide RNA hairpin loop found in Escherichia coli, r(UUAAGU). Biochemistry. 2001;**40**(33):9879-9886 [Internet]. [cited 2022 Jul 8]. Available from: https://pubs.acs.org/doi/abs/10.1021/bi011226x

[50] Al-Hashimi HM. NMR studies of nucleic acid dynamics. Journal of Magnetic Resonance. 2013;237:191. [Internet]. [cited 2022 Jul 8]. Available from: /pmc/articles/PMC3984477/

[51] Wang X, Alnabati E, Aderinwale TW, Maddhuri Venkata Subramaniya SR, Terashi G, Kihara D. Detecting protein and DNA/RNA structures in cryo-EM maps of intermediate resolution using deep learning. Nature Communications. 2021; **12**(1):1-9 [Internet]. [cited 2022 Jul 8]. Available from: https://www.nature.com/articles/s41467-021-22577-3

[52] Berman HM, Westbrook J, Feng Z, Gilliland G, Bhat TN, Weissig H, et al. The Protein Data Bank. Nucleic Acids Research. 2000;**28**(1):235-242 [Internet]. [cited 2022 Jul 8]. Available from: https://academic.oup.com/nar/article/28/1/235/2384399

[53] PDB Statistics: DNA-only Structures Released Per Year [Internet]. [cited 2022 Jul 8]. Available from: https://www.rcsb.org/stats/growth/growth-dna

[54] Feng Y, Yan Y, He J, Tao H, Wu Q, Huang SY. Docking and scoring for nucleic acid–ligand interactions: Principles and current status. Drug Discovery Today. 2022;**27**(3):838-847

[55] Sanderson BA, Sowersby DS, Crosby S, Goss M, Lewis LK, Beall GW. Charge density and particle size effects on oligonucleotide and plasmid DNA binding to nanosized hydrotalcite. Biointerphases. 2013;**8**(1):1-11 [Internet]. [cited 2022 Jul 10]. Available from: https://pubmed.ncbi.nlm.nih.gov/24706120/

[56] Bao L, Zhang X, Jin L, et al. Flexibility of nucleic acids: From DNA to RNA. Chinese Physics B. 2015;**25**(1): 018703 [Internet]. [cited 2022 Jul 10]. Available from: https://iopscience.iop.

org/article/10.1088/1674-1056/25/1/018703

[57] Mordor [Internet]. [cited 2022 Jul 10]. Available from: http://mondale.ucsf.edu/science/mordor.html.sav

[58] Stagno JR, Liu Y, Bhandari YR, Conrad CE, Panja S, Swain M, et al. Structures of riboswitch RNA reaction states by mix-and-inject XFEL serial crystallography. Nature. 2017;**541**(7636): 242-246 [Internet]. [cited 2022 Jul 10]. Available from: https://www.nature.com/articles/nature20599

[59] Lopéz-Blanco JR, Garzón JI, Chacón P. iMod: Multipurpose normal mode analysis in internal coordinates. Bioinformatics. 2011;**27**(20):2843-2850 [Internet]. [cited 2022 Jul 10]. Available from: https://academic.oup.com/bioinformatics/article/27/20/2843/202794

[60] Tessaro F, Scapozza L. How "Protein-Docking" Translates into the New Emerging Field of Docking Small Molecules to Nucleic Acids? Molecules. 2020;**25**(12):2749. DOI: 10.3390/molecules25122749. PMID: 32545835; PMCID: PMC7355999

[61] Guilbert C, James TL. Docking to RNA via root-Mean-Square-deviation-driven energy minimization with flexible ligands and flexible targets. Journal of Chemical Information and Modeling. 2008;**48**(6):1257-1268 [Internet]. [cited 2022 Jul 10]. Available from: http://pmc/articles/PMC2910576/

[62] Martella M, Pichiorri F, Chikhale RV, Abdelhamid MAS, Waller ZAE, Smith SS. i-motif formation and spontaneous deletions in human cells. Nucleic Acids Research. 2022;**50**(6, 55):3445 [Internet]. [cited 2022 Jul 10]. Available from: https://academic.oup.com/nar/article/50/6/3445/6543540

[63] King JJ, Irving KL, Evans CW, Chikhale RV, Becker R, Morris CJ, et al. DNA G-Quadruplex and i-motif structure formation is interdependent in human cells. Journal of the American Chemical Society. 2020;**142**(49): 20600-20604 [Internet]. [cited 2022 Jul 10]. Available from: https://pubs.acs.org/doi/abs/10.1021/jacs.0c11708

[64] Wang M, Yu Y, Liang C, Lu A, Zhang G. Recent Advances in Developing Small Molecules Targeting Nucleic Acid. International Journal of Molecular Sciences. 2016;**17**(6):779. DOI: 10.3390/ijms17060779. PMID: 27248995; PMCID: PMC4926330

[65] Krüger A, Zimbres FM, Kronenberger T, Wrenger C. Molecular modeling applied to nucleic acid-based molecule development. Biomolecules. 2018;**8**(3):83 [Internet]. [cited 2022 Jul 19]. Available from: https://www.mdpi.com/2218-273X/8/3/83/htm

[66] Holt PA, Chaires JB, Trent JO. Molecular Docking of Intercalators and Groove-Binders to Nucleic Acids Using Autodock and Surflex. [cited 2022 Jul 19]; Available from: https://pubs.acs.org/sharingguidelines

[67] Chikhale RV, Guneri D, Yuan R, Morris CJ, ZAE W. Identification of sugar-containing natural products that interact with i-motif DNA. Bioorganic & Medicinal Chemistry Letters. 2022;**73**:128886 [Internet]. [cited 2022 Jul 23]. Available from: https://linkinghub.elsevier.com/retrieve/pii/S0960894X22003626

[68] Katchalski-Katzir E, Shariv I, Eisenstein M, Friesem AA, Aflalo C, Vakser IA. Molecular surface recognition: Determination of geometric fit between proteins and their ligands by correlation techniques. Proceedings of the National Academy of Sciences of the United States of America. 1992;**89**(6):

2195-2199 [Internet]. [cited 2022 Jul 19]. Available from: https://www.pnas.org

[69] Gabb HA, Jackson RM, Sternberg MJE. Modelling protein docking using shape complementarity, electrostatics and biochemical information. Journal of Molecular Biology. 1997;**272**(1):106-120

[70] Carter P, Lesk VI, Islam SA, Sternberg MJE. Protein–protein docking using 3D-dock in rounds 3, 4, and 5 of CAPRI. Proteins: Structure, Function, and Bioinformatics. 2005; **60**(2):281-288 [Internet]. [cited 2022 Jul 19]. Available from: https://onlinelibrary.wiley.com/doi/full/10.1002/prot.20571

[71] Protein Docking using Spherical Polar Fourier Correlations [Internet]. [cited 2022 Jul 19]. Available from: https://onlinelibrary.wiley.com/doi/epdf/10.1002/%28SICI%291097-0134%2820000501%2939%3A2%3C178%3A%3AAID-PROT8%3E3.0.CO%3B2-6

[72] Roberts VA, Thompson EE, Pique ME, Perez MS, ten Eyck LF. DOT2: Macromolecular docking with improved biophysical models. Journal of Computational Chemistry. 2013;**34**(20): 1743-1758 [Internet]. [cited 2022 Jul 21]. Available from: https://pubmed.ncbi.nlm.nih.gov/23695987/

[73] Dominguez C, Boelens R, AMJJ B. HADDOCK: A protein-protein docking approach based on biochemical or biophysical information. Journal of the American Chemical Society. 2003; **125**(7):1731-1737 [Internet]. [cited 2022 Jul 21]. Available from: https://pubs.acs.org/doi/full/10.1021/ja026939x

[74] Schneidman-Duhovny D, Inbar Y, Nussinov R, Wolfson HJ. PatchDock and SymmDock: Servers for rigid and symmetric docking. Nucleic Acids Research. 2005;**33**(suppl_2):W363-W367 [Internet]. [cited 2022 Jul 21]. Available from: https://academic.oup.com/nar/article/33/suppl_2/W363/2505698

[75] Mashiach E, Schneidman-Duhovny D, Peri A, Shavit Y, Nussinov R, Wolfson HJ. An integrated suite of fast docking algorithms. Proteins: Structure, Function, and Bioinformatics. 2010;**78**(15): 3197-3204 [Internet]. [cited 2022 Jul 21]. Available from: https://onlinelibrary.wiley.com/doi/full/10.1002/prot.l22790

[76] Banitt I, Wolfson HJ. ParaDock: A flexible non-specific DNA—Rigid protein docking algorithm. Nucleic Acids Research. 2011;**39**(20):e135-e135 [Internet]. [cited 2022 Jul 21]. Available from: https://academic.oup.com/nar/article/39/20/e135/2409748

[77] Tuszynska I, Magnus M, Jonak K, Dawson W, Bujnicki JM. NPDock: A web server for protein–nucleic acid docking. Nucleic Acids Research. 2015;**43**(W1): W425-W430 [Internet]. [cited 2022 Jul 21]. Available from: https://academic.oup.com/nar/article/43/W1/W425/2467938

[78] Yan Y, Zhang D, Zhou P, Li B, Huang SY. HDOCK: A web server for protein–protein and protein–DNA/RNA docking based on a hybrid strategy. Nucleic Acids Research. 2017;**45**(W1): W365-W373 [Internet]. [cited 2022 Jul 21]. Available from: https://academic.oup.com/nar/article/45/W1/W365/3829194

[79] Jones G, Willett P, Glen RC, Leach AR, Taylor R. Development and validation of a genetic algorithm for flexible docking. Journal of Molecular Biology. 1997;**267**(3):727-748

[80] Pfeffer P, Gohlke H. DrugScore RNA - knowledge-based scoring

function to predict RNA - ligand interactions. Journal of Chemical Information and Modeling. 2007;**47**(5): 1868-1876 [Internet]. [cited 2022 Jul 27]. Available from: https://pubs.acs.org/doi/full/10.1021/ci700134p

[81] Trott O, Olson AJ. AutoDock Vina: Improving the speed and accuracy of docking with a new scoring function, efficient optimization, and multithreading. Journal of Computational Chemistry. 2010;**31**(2): 455-461 [Internet]. [cited 2022 Jul 21]. Available from: https://onlinelibrary.wiley.com/doi/full/10.1002/jcc.21334

[82] Morris GM, Ruth H, Lindstrom W, Sanner MF, Belew RK, Goodsell DS, et al. AutoDock4 and AutoDockTools4: Automated docking with selective receptor flexibility. Journal of Computational Chemistry. 2009;**30**(16): 2785. [Internet]. [cited 2022 Jul 21]. Available from: /pmc/articles/PMC2760638/

[83] Morris GM, Goodsell DS, Huey R, Olson AJ. Distributed automated docking of flexible ligands to proteins: Parallel applications of AutoDock 2.4. Journal of Computer-Aided Molecular Design. 1996;**10**(4):293-304 [Internet]. [cited 2022 Jul 21]. Available from: https://pubmed.ncbi.nlm.nih.gov/8877701/

[84] Goodsell DS, Olson AJ. Automated docking of substrates to proteins by simulated annealing. Proteins. 1990; **8**(3):195-202 [Internet]. [cited 2022 Jul 21]. Available from: https://pubmed.ncbi.nlm.nih.gov/2281083/

[85] Jain AN. Surflex: Fully automatic flexible molecular docking using a molecular similarity-based search engine. Journal of Medicinal Chemistry. 2003;**46**(4):499-511 [Internet]. [cited 2022 Jul 21]. Available from: https://pubmed.ncbi.nlm.nih.gov/12570372/

[86] Ruiz-Carmona S, Alvarez-Garcia D, Foloppe N, Garmendia-Doval AB, Juhos S. rDock: A fast, versatile and open source program for docking ligands to proteins and nucleic acids. PLoS Computational Biology. 2014;**10**(4): 1003571 [Internet]. [cited 2022 Jul 22]. Available from: www.ploscompbiol.org

[87] Feng Y, Zhang K, Wu Q, Huang SY. NLDock: A fast nucleic acid–ligand docking algorithm for modeling RNA/DNA–ligand complexes. Journal of Chemical Information and Modeling. 2021;**61**:4771-4782. [Internet]. [cited 2022 Jul 21]. DOI: 10.1021/acs.jcim.1c00341

[88] Feng Y, Huang S. ITScore-NL: An Iterative Knowledge-Based Scoring Function for Nucleic Acid-Ligand Interactions. Journal of Chemical Information and Modeling. 2020;**60**(12): 6698-6708

[89] Philips A, Milanowska K, Łach G, Bujnicki JM. LigandRNA: Computational predictor of RNA–ligand interactions. RNA. 2013;**19**(12):1605-1616 [Internet]. [cited 2022 Jul 22]. Available from: http://rnajournal.cshlp.org/content/19/12/1605.full

[90] Lang PT, Brozell SR, Mukherjee S, Pettersen EF, Meng EC, Thomas V, et al. DOCK 6: Combining techniques to model RNA-small molecule complexes. RNA. 2009;**15**(6):1219-1230 [Internet]. [cited 2022 Jul 22]. Available from: https://pubmed.ncbi.nlm.nih.gov/19369428/

[91] Aminpour M, Montemagno C, Tuszynski JA. An Overview of Molecular Modeling for Drug Discovery with Specific Illustrative Examples of Applications. Molecules. 2019;**24**(9):

1693. DOI: 10.3390/molecules24091693. PMID: 31052253; PMCID: PMC6539951

[92] Bentham Science Publisher BSP. Scoring functions for protein-ligand docking. Current Protein & Peptide Science. 2006;7(5):407-420

[93] Li J, Fu A, Zhang L. An Overview of Scoring Functions Used for Protein-Ligand Interactions in Molecular Docking. Interdisciplinary Sciences. 2019;**11**(2):320-328. DOI: 10.1007/s12539-019-00327-w. Epub 2019 Mar 15. PMID: 30877639

[94] Meli R, Morris GM, Biggin PC. Scoring functions for protein-ligand binding affinity prediction using structure-based deep learning: A review. Frontiers in Bioinformatics. 2022;**2**

[95] Adcock SA, McCammon JA. Molecular dynamics: Survey of methods for simulating the activity of proteins. Chemical Reviews. 2006;**106**(5):1589-1615

[96] Ain QU, Aleksandrova A, Roessler FD, Ballester PJ. Machine-learning scoring functions to improve structure-based binding affinity prediction and virtual screening. Wiley Interdisciplinary Reviews: Computational Molecular Science. 2015;**5**(6):405-424. DOI: 10.1002/wcms.1225. Epub 2015 Aug 28. PMID: 27110292; PMCID: PMC4832270

[97] Guedes IA, Pereira FSS, Dardenne LE. Empirical ScoringFunctions for Structure-Based VirtualScreening: Applications, CriticalAspects, and Challenges. Frontiers in Pharmacology. 2018;**9**:1089

[98] Fujimoto KJ, Minami S, Yanai T. Machine-learning- and knowledge-based scoring functions incorporating ligand and protein fingerprints. ACS Omega. 2022;**7**(22):19030-19039

[99] Stefaniak F, Bujnicki JM. AnnapuRNA: A scoring function for predicting RNA-small molecule binding poses. PLoS Computational Biology. 2021;**17**(2):e1008309. DOI: 10.1371/journal.pcbi.1008309. PMID: 33524009; PMCID: PMC7877745

[100] Ruiz-Carmona S, Alvarez-Garcia D, Foloppe N, Garmendia-Doval AB, Juhos S, Schmidtke P, et al. rDock: A fast, versatile and open source program for docking ligands to proteins and nucleic acids. PLoS Computational Biology. 2014;**10**(4):1-7

[101] Morley SD, Afshar M. Validation of an empirical RNA-ligand scoring function for fast flexible docking using Ribodock. Journal of Computer-Aided Molecular Design. 2004;**18**(3):189-208

[102] Kollman PA, Massova I, Reyes C, Kuhn B, Huo S, Chong L, et al. Calculating structures and free energies of complex molecules: Combining molecular mechanics and continuum models. Accounts of Chemical Research. 2000;**33**(12):889-897

[103] Genheden S, Ryde U. The MM/PBSA and MM/GBSA methods to estimate ligand-binding affinities. Expert Opinion on Drug Discovery. 2015;**10**(5):449-461

[104] Aamir M, Singh VK, Dubey MK, Meena M, Kashyap SP, Katari SK, et al. In silico prediction, characterization, molecular docking, and dynamic studies on fungal SDRs as novel targets for searching potential fungicides against fusarium wilt in tomato. Frontiers in Pharmacology. 2018;**9**(OCT):1038

[105] UCSF. Flexible Docking with MORDOR [Internet]. [cited 2022 Jul 31].

Available from: http://mondale.ucsf.edu/index_mordor.html

[106] Jiang Y, Chen SJ. RLDOCK method for predicting RNA-small molecule binding modes. Methods. 2022;**197** (January 2021):97-105

[107] Zhou Y, Jiang Y, Chen SJ. RNA–ligand molecular docking: Advances and challenges. Wiley Interdisciplinary Reviews: Computational Molecular Science. 2022;**12**(3):1-32

[108] Sousa SF, Fernandes PA, Ramos MJ. Protein-ligand docking: Current status and future challenges. Proteins. 2006; **65**(1):15-26

[109] Ballester PJ, Mitchell JBO. A machine learning approach to predicting protein–ligand binding affinity with applications to molecular docking. Bioinformatics. 2010;**26**(9):1169-1175 [Internet]. [cited 2022 Jul 28]. Available from: https://academic.oup.com/bioinformatics/article/26/9/1169/199938

[110] Nguyen DD, Wei GW. AGL-score: Algebraic graph learning score for protein-ligand binding scoring, ranking, docking, and screening. Journal of Chemical Information and Modeling. 2019;**59**(7):3291-3304 [Internet]. [cited 2022 Jul 28]. Available from: https://pubs.acs.org/doi/full/10.1021/acs.jcim.9b00334

[111] Li L, Wang B, Meroueh SO. Support vector regression scoring of receptor-ligand complexes for rank-ordering and virtual screening of chemical libraries. Journal of Chemical Information and Modeling. 2011;**51**(9):2132-2138 [Internet]. [cited 2022 Jul 28]. Available from: https://pubs.acs.org/doi/full/10.1021/ci200078f

[112] Durrant JD, Friedman AJ, Rogers KE, McCammon JA. Comparing neural-network scoring functions and the state of the art: Applications to common library screening. Journal of Chemical Information and Modeling. 2013;**53**(7):1726-1735 [Internet]. [cited 2022 Jul 28]. Available from: https://pubs.acs.org/doi/full/10.1021/ci400042y

[113] Jiménez J, Doerr S, Martínez-Rosell G, Rose AS, de Fabritiis G. DeepSite: Protein-binding site predictor using 3D-convolutional neural networks. Bioinformatics. 2017;**33**(19):3036-3042 [Internet]. [cited 2022 Jul 28]. Available from: https://academic.oup.com/bioinformatics/article/33/19/3036/3859178

[114] Lim J, Ryu S, Park K, Choe YJ, Ham J, Kim WY. Predicting drug-target interaction using a novel graph neural network with 3D structure-embedded graph representation. Journal of Chemical Information and Modeling. 2019;**59**(9):3981-3988 [Internet]. [cited 2022 Jul 28]. Available from: https://pubs.acs.org/doi/full/10.1021/acs.jcim.9b00387

[115] Chhabra S, Xie J, Frank AT. RNAPosers: Machine learning classifiers for ribonucleic acid-ligand poses. Journal of Physical Chemistry B. 2020;**124**(22):4436-4445 [Internet]. [cited 2022 Jul 27]. Available from: https://pubs.acs.org/doi/full/10.1021/acs.jpcb.0c02322

[116] Stefaniak F, Bujnicki JM. AnnapuRNA: A scoring function for predicting RNA-small molecule binding poses. PLoS Computational Biology. 2021;**17**(2):e1008309 [Internet]. [cited 2022 Jul 29]. Available from: https://journals.plos.org/ploscompbiol/article?id=10.1371/journal.pcbi.1008309

Chapter 6

Repurposing Drugs as Potential Therapeutics for the SARS-Cov-2 Viral Infection: Automatizing a Blind Molecular Docking High-throughput Pipeline

Aldo Herrera-Rodulfo, Mariana Andrade-Medina and Mauricio Carrillo-Tripp

Abstract

In the context of the COVID-19 pandemic, scientists worldwide have been looking for ways to stop it using different approaches. One strategy is to look among drugs that have already proved safe for use in humans and tested for other illnesses. Several components from the virus and the infected cell are the potential therapeutic targets from a molecular perspective. We explain how we implemented a cavity-guided blind molecular docking algorithm into a high-throughput computational pipeline to automatically screen and analyze a large set of drugs over a group of SARS-CoV-2 and cell proteins involved in the infection process. We discuss the need to significantly extend the conformational space sampling to find an accurate target-ligand complex. Our results identify nine drugs with potential multi-target activity against COVID-19 at different stages of the infection and immune system evasion. These results are relevant in understanding the SARS-CoV-2 drug's molecular mechanisms and further clinical treatment development. The code developed is available on GitHub [https://github.com/tripplab/HTVS].

Keywords: SARS-CoV-2, COVID-19, drug repurposing, cavity-guided blind molecular docking, high-throughput virtual screening

1. Introduction

The coronavirus disease-2019 (COVID-19) is the third documented viral outbreak caused by a member of the *Coronaviridae* family. From 2002 to 2004, the severe acute respiratory syndrome coronavirus (SARS-CoV) spread to 29 countries, causing 8422 confirmed cases and 916 deaths, and is considered the first emerging epidemic of the twenty-first century [1, 2]. Later in 2012, the middle-east respiratory syndrome coronavirus (MERS-CoV) caused 2585 confirmed cases and 890 deaths to date [3]. In less than two decades since the appearance of SARS-CoV, the severe acute respiratory syndrome coronavirus 2 (SARS-CoV-2) emerged in late 2019 and has spread worldwide ever since by human-to-human transmission. As of April 29, 2022, there are more than 510 million confirmed cases and 6.2 million deaths related to SARS-CoV-2 infection, and it continues to increase at present [4]. The *Coronaviridae* family comprises a group of enveloped crown-shaped single-stranded positive-sensed RNA viruses (ssRNA+) with multiple domestic and wild animal reservoirs [5]. Lessons from previous and current outbreaks have shown the severity of cross-species transmission, which has led to concerns about health emergencies, such as COVID-19. The transmission of this disease occurs through an infected person's respiratory droplets carrying the SARS-CoV-2, and the severity ranges from asymptomatic cases, mild and moderate flu-like symptoms, to critical illness requiring intensive care with mechanical ventilation, and death [6]. Global contributions and efforts following the COVID-19 outbreak have unraveled a considerable amount of information about viral infection, transmission, infection cycles, and immune evasion. Currently, the three-dimensional proteome structures of the SARS-CoV-2 are available on the RCSB protein data bank [7]. Therefore, it is feasible to evaluate drug-like small molecules against relevant targets in the viral infection cycle through a structure-based molecular docking approach. Blind molecular docking, unlike traditional molecular docking, does not require prior knowledge of target binding sites, which simplifies the automatizing of the process since it only needs the structural information of the target. In the past, this process was considered less accurate than the traditional. However, methods, such as CB-dock, have overcome this limitation by reducing the nonrelevant conformation sampling by directing the molecular docking on putative sites instead of the whole protein structure [8]. The integration of this tool into our customized high-throughput virtual screening pipeline allows the screening of N sorted-by-size cavities. The cavity-based search is an exciting scenario because protein-ligand interactions usually occur in large protein cavities or pockets that frequently contain the active site [9]. Moreover, the exploration of cavities in the vicinity of protein-protein interfaces (PPI) is also an attractive approach to searching for effective inhibitors since it plays an essential role in nearly all biological processes, including SARS-CoV-2 infection [10, 11]. In this context, screening already-known drugs with described pharmacology, dose, toxicity, formulation, and proven to be safe for use in humans represents a low-risk and cost-effective strategy to considerably shorten the time required for drug approval [12, 13]. We present an in-house customizable pipeline that integrates a cavity-guided blind molecular docking algorithm to extend the conformation space sampling on putative sites significantly. We also report the methodology to follow and results of the virtual screening of 47 drugs for potential repurposing against 16 structures of 10 viral and cell targets that are key in the SARS-CoV-2 infection cycle.

2. Overview of the SARS-CoV-2 infection cycle

The initial stage of the infection cycle starts with the recognition and anchoring of the SARS-CoV-2 spike protein complex into the host angiotensin-converting enzyme 2 (ACE2) through the receptor-binding domain (RBD) located at each one of the 3S proteins [14]. Then, the activation of the spike occurs at the surface or endosome level by transmembrane serine protease 2 (TMPRSS2) or cathepsin B/L proteases, respectively, to allow viral entry [15]. Once the virus membrane merges with the cell membrane, the genomic material enters the cell. The cell's ribosomes then translate the viral RNA into pp1a/ab polyproteins, which will be later processed by cleavage through the enzymatic activity of the main protease (Mpro) and the papain-like protease (PLpro) [16]. This process will release 16 non-structural proteins (NSPs), including the RNA-dependent RNA polymerase (NSP12) and co-factors NSP7, and NSP8 of the RNA-replication machinery (Rdrp). After replication, expression of the structural proteins occurs, the genomic material is packaged, and the virion is assembled on a lipid membrane and matured for subsequent exocytosis. In addition, evidence suggests that the SARS-CoV-2 proteases and some of their cleavage products, besides their critical function for the proper infection process, interplay with the host's innate immune response through different mechanisms [17]. In particular, PLpro-ISG15 interaction allows the virus to evade the innate immune response through deubiquitination and deISGylation activities of the protease [18, 19]. Interestingly, the process occurs at the same binding cavity as the PLpro known inhibitor, GRL0617 [20].

3. Methods

The code for the cavity-detection guided blind docking (CB-Dock) [8] stand-alone version is freely available at Yang Cao's Lab webpage [http://clab.labshare.cn/cb-dock/php/manual.php#download].

The customized high-throughput virtual screening pipeline we developed can be accessed at GitHub [https://github.com/tripplab/HTVS].

3.1 Drug selection and modeling

We conducted an extensive scientific literature search for drugs reported as potentially able to prevent SARS-CoV-2 infection. The search included *in silico*, *in vitro*, and *in vivo* studies, covering different stages of the viral cycle. We grouped the reported ligands into five sets: the fusion and viral entry into the host cell (RPA), the polyprotein processing by viral proteases (RPB and RPD), the RNA replication machinery (RPC), and other drugs with alternative or unknown mechanisms (EXT).

We performed the molecular *in silico* modeling of each ligand's configuration using the PubChem compound identifier (CID) or, in its absence, using UCSF chimera 1.15 from scratch [21]. The solvent, ions, and other small molecules were removed in all cases, while charges and hydrogens were fixed at neutral pH. Then, ligands were subjected to energy minimization by 10,000 steepest descent steps and 1000 conjugate gradient steps to ensure the proper molecular conformation, saving the final structure in MOL2 format. The next step was to generate the files in PDBqt format using AutoDock Tools, considering the torsional degrees of freedom [22]. We used the PDBqt and MOL2 files as input for the high-throughput virtual screening pipeline. A list of all the ligands studied in this work is shown in **Table 1**.

3.2 Target selection and modeling

We included viral and cellular targets involved in the SARS-CoV-2 infection cycle, covering the entry, polyprotein processing, and replication. The targets' three-dimensional structures were obtained from the Research Collaboratory for Structural Bioinformatics Protein Data Bank (RCSB) in PDB format [65]. The complete structure of the spike homotrimer complex (PDB: 6VXX-1-1-1) was retrieved from the CHARMM-GUI Archive-COVID-19 proteins library [66]. We took special consideration to the spike complex given its large size and quaternary structure. We focused

ID	Drug	CID[a]	References
RPA01	Losartan	3961	[23, 24]
RPA02	Telmisartan	65,999	[23, 25]
RPA03	Arbidol	131,411	[26, 27]
RPA04	Camostat mesylate	5,284,360	[26, 28]
RPA05	Rimantadine	5071	[29]
RPA06	Chloroquine	2719	[26, 30]
RPA07	Hydroxychloroquine	3652	[26, 30]
RPA08	Baricitinib	44,205,240	[31, 32]
RPA09	Colchicine	6167	[33, 34]
RPA10	Disulfiram	3117	[35, 36]
RPA11	Ebselen	3194	[35–37]
RPA12	Hesperidin	10,621	[38, 39]
RPA13	Qingdainone	3,035,728	[40]
RPA14	Nafamostat	4413	[41, 42]
RPA15	Dipeptidyl nitrile-derivative	Compound 10	[43]
RPB01	Lopinavir	92,727	[26, 44]
RPB02	Ritonavir	392,622	[26, 44]
RPB03	Darunavir	213,039	[29, 45]
RPB04	Cobicistat	25,151,504	[45]
RPB05	Isatin-derivative	Compound 26	[46]
RPB06	Rupinatrivir	6,440,352	[47, 48]
RPB07	E-64	123,985	[49]
RPB08	N3 inhibitor	405,067,310	[50]
RPC01	Ribavirin	37,542	[51, 52]
RPC02	Sofosbuvir	45,375,808	[51, 52]
RPC03	Molnupiravir	145,996,610	[51, 52]
RPC04	Nilotinib	644,241	[53–55]
RPC05	Saquinavir	441,243	[29, 51, 52, 55]
RPC06	Tipranavir	54,682,461	[51, 52, 55]
RPC07	Lonafarnib	148,195	[55]
RPC08	Tegobuvir	23,649,154	[51, 52, 55]
RPC09	Simeprevir	24,873,435	[51, 52]
RPC10	Filibuvir	54,708,673	[51, 52, 55]
RPC11	Cepharanthine	10,206	[55]
RPC12	Redemsivir	121,304,016	[26, 51, 52]
RPC13	Favipiravir	492,405	[26, 51, 52]
RPD01	rac5c	76,853,649	[19]
EXT01	Ascorbic Acid	54,670,067	[56]

ID	Drug	CID[a]	References
EXT02	Ergocalciferol	5,280,793	[57, 58]
EXT03	Cholecalciferol	5,280,795	[57, 58]
EXT04	Ivermectin	6,321,424	[59]
EXT05	Azithromycin	447,043	[60]
EXT06	Heparin	772	[61]
EXT07	Methylprednisolone	6741	[62]
EXT08	Carvacrol	10,364	[63]
EXT09	Ursolic acid	45,358,157	[64]
EXT10	Oleanolic acid	485,707	[64]

[a]*In the absence of the CID, the reference to the original investigation and the compound number are provided.*

Table 1.
Ligand information, CID number, and reference of 47 drugs with potential activity against the SARS-CoV-2 viral cycle.

on four independent spike-based structures to extend the cavity sampling: the full-length spike's homotrimer complex, the homotrimer head (S1), 1 S protein monomer, and one isolated receptor-binding domain (RBD).

Water, ions, glycosylations, and co-crystallized ligands were removed from all targets. Charges and hydrogens were fixed at neutral pH using chimera 1.15, their structure optimized, and the final configuration saved in PDB format [21]. In total, 16 structures of 10 targets were curated, as summarized in **Table 2**.

3.3 Extended conformational space sampling maximizes the prediction accuracy of the target-ligand complex

Molecular docking is a computational method that allows to sample the conformational space and rank the ligand poses through an energy scoring function. It attempts to generate an optimized target-ligand complex conformation with the lowest binding free-energy change estimate, predicting the interaction of the two molecules in the energy minimum. This task is a cyclic process performed by systematic or stochastic search methods. However, the latter is the choice of preference since it increases the probability of finding an energetic global minimum conformation because the search initiates from different random points [78]. For this reason, the results of two or more molecular docking cycles are not necessarily the same due to the random nature of the conformational search method. Therefore, performing as many cycles as necessary to get as close as possible to the energetic global minimum conformation is essential.

Easy customization of this parameter in the developed high-throughput virtual screening code offers the user the possibility of an exhaustive sampling of the conformational space that maximizes the accuracy of target-ligand complex prediction.

3.4 High-throughput virtual screening pipeline

We have developed in-house bash scripts that integrate the CB-Dock's cavity-guided blind molecular docking method, which automatically identifies binding sites by calculating putative cavities through a curvature-based detection approach. Molecular

ID	Target	PDB ID[a]	SARS-CoV-2 infection step	References
H00	ACE2	1R4L_A	Viral recognition	[67]
H01	ACE2 (B0AT1 closed complex)	6M18_B	Viral recognition	[68]
H02	ACE2 (B0AT1 open complex)	6M1D_B	Viral recognition	[68]
H03	TMPRSS2	7MEQ_A	Viral priming	[69]
H04	Cathepsin B	3AI8_B	Viral priming	[70]
H05	Cathepsin L	2NQD_B	Viral priming	[71]
V01	Spike homotrimer	6VXX1-1-1	Viral recognition	[72, 73]
V01H	Spike homotrimer head	6VXX1-1-1	Viral recognition	[72, 73]
V02	S protein	6VXX1-1-1	Viral recognition	[72, 73]
V02R	S protein's RBD	6VXX1-1-1	Viral recognition	[72, 73]
V03	Mpro	6LU7_A	Polyprotein processing	[74]
V08	PLpro	7JRN_A	Polyprotein processing	[20]
V04	NSP12	7AAP_A	RNA replication	[75]
V05	NSP7	6M71_C	RNA replication	[76]
V06	NSP8	6NUR_B	RNA replication	[77]
V07	Rdrp-complex (NSP12-NSP7-NSP8)	6M71_ABC	RNA replication	[76]

[a]*Underscore denotes the chain selected from PDB coordinates files.*

Table 2.
Structural information and PDB entries of viral (V) and host (H) targets included.

docking analysis is conducted in these putative cavities to sample and rank ligand poses and estimate the best target-ligand complex binding energy scores per cycle.

The pipeline has three phases comprised of nested loops, schematized in **Figure 1** as a flowchart. First, each target T is subject to a cavity detection step based on a spatial geometry measure of curvature distribution on the protein surface [79]. Cavity identification is achieved by clustering the resulting surface points by density and curvature factor [80]. All cavities are then sorted by size, considering their solvent-accessible surface area. Second, the algorithm automatically configures a docking box for each cavity by defining its center and size, considering the cavity space location and the ligand L size. Finally, in the third step, the blind molecular docking is performed by the AutoDock VINA algorithm [8, 81] for the user-defined top N cavities for each ligand L and each target T. This protocol will be repeated for K-independent rounds.

In our study, we found that the optimal number of independent rounds is $K = 30$ since it is at this point that the conformational search converges to the lowest energy binding pose; that is, more rounds do not improve the prediction. The calculations were performed on the top $N = 10$ cavities for each $T - L$ pair to significantly extend the cavity and conformational space sampling. The value of these parameters is easily customizable at the top section of the bash script.

3.5 Target-ligand co-crystallization complex prediction

The method we used for automatizing the virtual high-throughput screening process is blind; that is, it does not require any information on the binding site. Hence, we

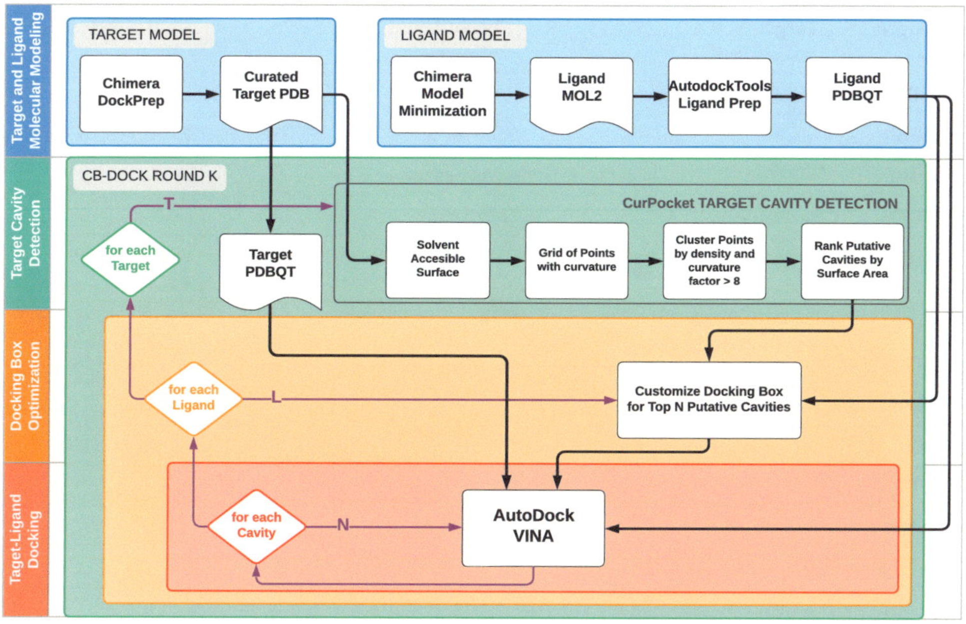

Figure 1.
Flowchart of the customized high-throughput virtual screening pipeline implemented in this work. Four phases are involved, i) target and ligand molecular modeling (blue), ii) target cavity detection (green), iii) docking box optimization (orange), and iv) target-ligand docking (red).

validated its predictions by reproducing the enzymatic targets' experimental binding complexes. We gathered a set of ligands with available complex co-crystallized data. Eight known enzymatic inhibitors were modeled, optimized, and evaluated under the same methodology conditions as the rest of the ligands included in this study. The ligands in the control set are listed in **Table 3**.

Furthermore, at this time, a small drug-like co-crystallized molecule in complex with the spike homotrimer does not yet exist. We included amantadine (INV05) in our set as a negative control since it inhibits the SARS-CoV-2 infection but does not prevent spike-ACE2 interaction [83].

3.6 Data analysis and selection criteria

We inspected the top 10 size-ranked putative cavity sites screened for each target. We selected those that either had the active site (targets ACE2, TMPRSS2, cathepsin B/L, Mpro, and NSP12), or were inside a quaternary interface (targets spike, PLpro, and Rdrp). We selected the $T - L$ complex conformation with the best affinity estimation, that is, the conformation with the lowest energy scores after $K = 30$ independent rounds for each target-ligand pair. We organized the data in matrix form and analyzed it with the statistical R package function *heatmap.2*. Rows (ligands) or columns (targets) were scaled to have average = 0 and standard deviation = 1 and generated a Z-score heatmap representation. Finally, we identified potential drugs for repurposing as those ligands with the best energy score estimate at least one standard deviation away from the mean toward more negative values. The data matrix of the VINA scores of the conformation with the lowest scores after $K = 30$ independent

Target ID	Target name	Ligand	PDB ID	Reference
1. Co-crystallized reproducibility				
INH01	ACE2	MLN-4760	1R4L	[67]
INH02	TMPRSS2	4-Guanidinobenzoic acid	7MEQ	[69]
INH03	Cathepsin B	Nitroxoline	3AI8	[70]
INH04	Cathepsin L	4-Bipheylacetyl-cys-(D)-ARG-TYR -N-(2-Phenylethyl) Amide	2NQD	[71]
INV01	Mpro	Narlaprevir	7JYC	[20]
INV02	NSP12	Remdesivir	7BV2	[82]
INV03	NSP12	Favipiravir	7AAP	[75]
INV04	PLpro	GRL0617	7JRN	[20]
2. Negative control[a]				
INV05	Spike	Amantadine	NA	[83]

[a]*Does not prevent ACE2-Spike interaction despite inhibiting* in vitro *SARS-CoV-2 replication.*

Table 3.
Modeled ligands to validate that the method is capable of reproducing the co-crystallized complex conformations and previous in vitro *findings (negative control).*

cycles of each target-ligand pair for known inhibitors and the set of ligands evaluated are provided in the appendix section as **Tables A-1** and **A-2**.

4. Results

4.1 Blind docking correctly reproduces co-crystallized known-inhibitor binding

We found that the $T - L$ complex conformation with the lowest energy for the known co-crystallized inhibitors in our control set successfully reproduces the ligand binding at the active site with an RMSD below 1 Å in most cases, as shown in **Figure 2**. These findings strongly suggest that the implemented high-throughput blind docking cavity-guided protocol can accurately predict the binding mode of the $T - L$ data in the experimental set.

4.2 Statistical analysis of the data: Sorting results by target

After doing all the blind docking calculations with an extended conformation sampling, we analyzed the most negative energy scores. We performed a Z-score transformation of the data for each independent column in the matrix (targets T). The graphical representation of the results is shown as a heatmap in **Figure 3** using a six-color code based on the Z-score value.

Since each column gathers the results for a different target, it is thus possible to identify which ligands had the best scores for each target (in green). It is worth noting that cathepsin L (H05) and PLpro (V08) co-crystallized inhibitors give a good binding free-energy estimate. Most of the co-crystallized inhibitors remained near the mean

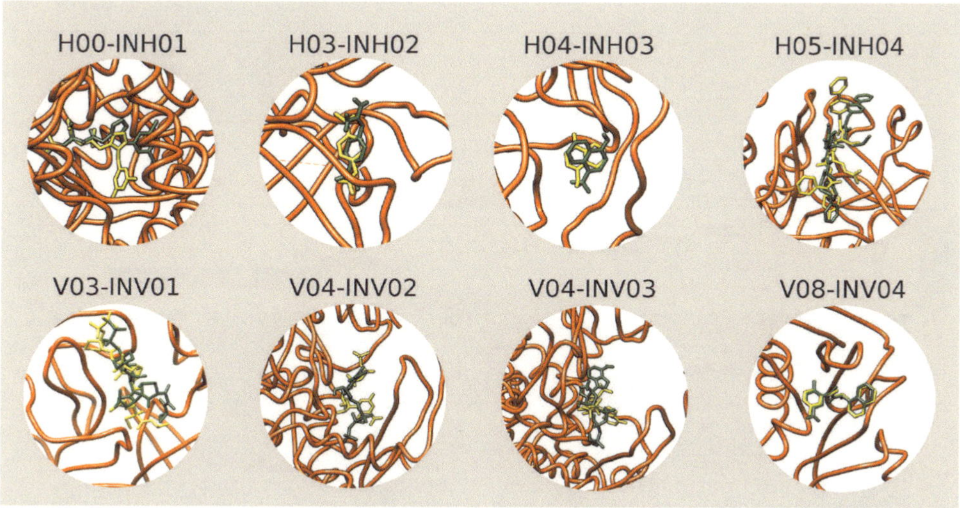

Figure 2.
Target-ligand complex superimposition of native co-crystallized inhibitors (yellow) and the best-predicted ligand conformation after $K = 30$ independent blind docking pipeline rounds (green). The molecular targets (orange) are ACE2 labeled as H00, TMPRSS2 (H03), cathepsin B (H04), cathepsin L (H05), Mpro (V03), NSP12 (V04), and PLpro (V08), created with the visual molecular dynamics (VMD) [84].

(in black, with respect to the experimental drug set), except for amantadine (INV05), which presents a positive Z-score value for the spike's RBD (in red). The latter is concomitant to previous works, where amantadine fails to prevent the spike-ACE2 quaternary interaction [83].

4.3 Nine ligands showed potential for drug repurposing against targets involved in SARS-CoV-2 infection

Out of the 47 drugs screened, nine showed potential inhibition against viral or host targets of the SARS-CoV-2 infection cycle. Saquinavir, simeprevir, nilotinib, an isatin-derivative, telmisartan, tegobuvir, qingdainone, rac5c, and nafamostat achieved the selection criteria. Interestingly, all but rac5c and nafamostat showed the best scores against more than one target. The schematic representation of these results is summarized in **Table 4**.

4.4 Sorting results by ligand: The screened ligands showed a preference for ACE2, Spike, and PLpro targets

Also, we inspected the results by ligand, performing a Z-score analysis by row (ligands). Since the rows gather data from the $L - T$ complex, it is thus possible to identify which ligand had the best scores on any particular target, that is, which target T might be a potential pharmacological target for the ligand L. The results are presented in **Figure 4** with a heatmap, using the same color-based code as previously described (see Section 4.2). The targets having most of the ligands in the experimental set with a negative Z-score are ACE2 H00, H01, and H02, and the spike protein structures V01, V01H, and V02 (see **Table 2**). The results suggest a greater acceptance of those two targets for the ligands as drug-like molecules, at least in the cavities

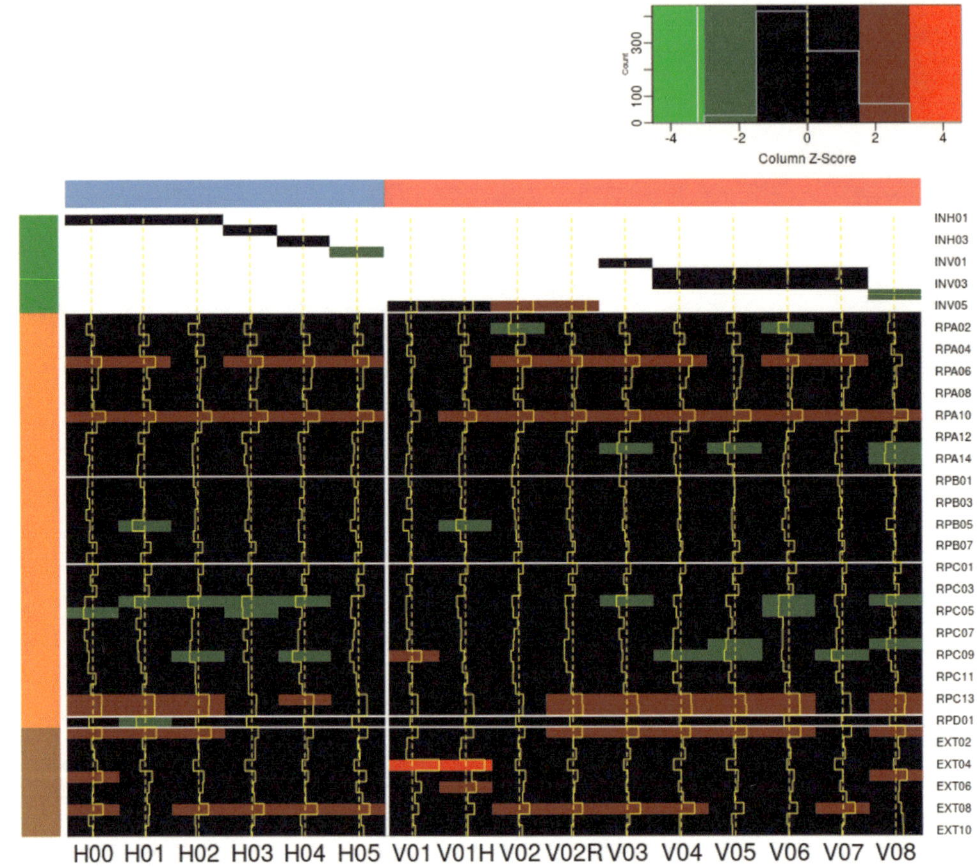

Figure 3.
*Target (columns) and ligand (rows) complex docking results. Heatmap of binding free-energy change estimates, using a color-based code according to the Z-score value through column analysis. Targets are grouped as host proteins (blue) and virus proteins (pink). Ligands are grouped by control set (green), potential repurposing drugs (orange), and others (brown). IDs correspond to those defined in **Tables 1–3**. Black shades represent ligands around the set's mean. In green shades, ligands with at least one negative standard deviation from the mean. Red shades represent ligands with at least one positive standard deviation from the mean.*

evaluated. These findings are not a minor fact because those targets are directly involved in the first step of the viral infection.

The ligands such as arbidol, colchicine, qingdainone, nafamostat, and carvacrol exhibit a binding preference to PLpro (V08). It is important to highlight the essential function of the protease PLpro for processing the viral proteome and evading the host's innate immune system. In the latter case, PLpro cleaves off post-translational modifications, such as ubiquitin and ubiquitin-like proteins from cell proteins, disrupting the inflammatory signaling pathway necessary for an appropriate immune response [18, 85]. Noteworthy, the potential PLpro inhibitors we have identified in the present work as repurposed drugs form a $T - L$ complex in the cavity where GRL0617 binds, located in the USP domain [20]. The inhibition of this site means blocking the interaction with the ubiquitin-like protein ISG15, evading the immune mechanisms and compromising its canonical enzymatic activity due to the proximity of the assessed site to the active site.

ID	Drug	Target	VINA score	Z-score[a]
RPC05	Saquinavir	ACE2 (H00)	−12.9	−1.70
RPB05	Isatin-derivative	ACE2 (H01)	−10.7	−2.06
RPC04	Nilotinib		−10.2	−1.72
RPD01	rac5c		−9.9	−1.51
RPC04	Nilotinib	ACE2 (H02)	−10.7	−1.85
RPC09	Simeprevir		−10.4	−1.62
RPC04	Nilotinib	TMPRSS2 (H03)	−8.9	−1.58
RPC05	Saquinavir		−8.8	−1.49
RPC04	Nilotinib	Cathepsin B (H04)	−9.6	−1.64
RPC09	Simeprevir		−10.3	−2.20
RPA02	Telmisartan	Spike (V02)	−9.4	−1.63
RPB05	Isatin-derivative	Spike (V01H)	−10.9	−1.67
RPA13	Qingdainone	Mpro (V03)	−9.4	−1.56
RPC04	Nilotinib		−9.7	−1.80
RPC09	Simeprevir	NSP12 (V04)	−9.1	−1.60
RPA13	Qingdainone	NSP7 (V05)	−7.4	−1.69
RPC08	Tegobuvir		−7.3	−1.59
RPC09	Simeprevir		−7.6	−1.89
RPA02	Telmisartan	NSP8 (V06)	−8.8	−1.65
RPC04	Nilotinib		−8.9	−1.73
RPC05	Saquinavir		−9	−1.80
RPC09	Simeprevir	Rdrp (V07)	−10	−1.96
RPA13	Qingdainone	PLpro (V08)	−9.9	−1.72
RPA14	Nafamostat		−10.1	−1.88
RPC04	Nilotinib		−9.8	−1.65
RPC08	Tegobuvir		−9.8	−1.65

[a]*Z-scores were calculated by the target.*

Table 4.
Potential drugs for repurposing with the most negative free-energy change score found and their corresponding Z-score value grouped by the target.

5. Scientific evidence to support our findings

5.1 Saquinavir and simeprevir targeting viral entry and Rdrp quaternary complex formation

Saquinavir is a peptide-mimetic HIV inhibitor. However, some reports suggest potential inhibitory activity against SARS-CoV-2 proteases [86–88] and other targets involved in the viral infection, such as the Rdrp replication complex [55, 89] and the

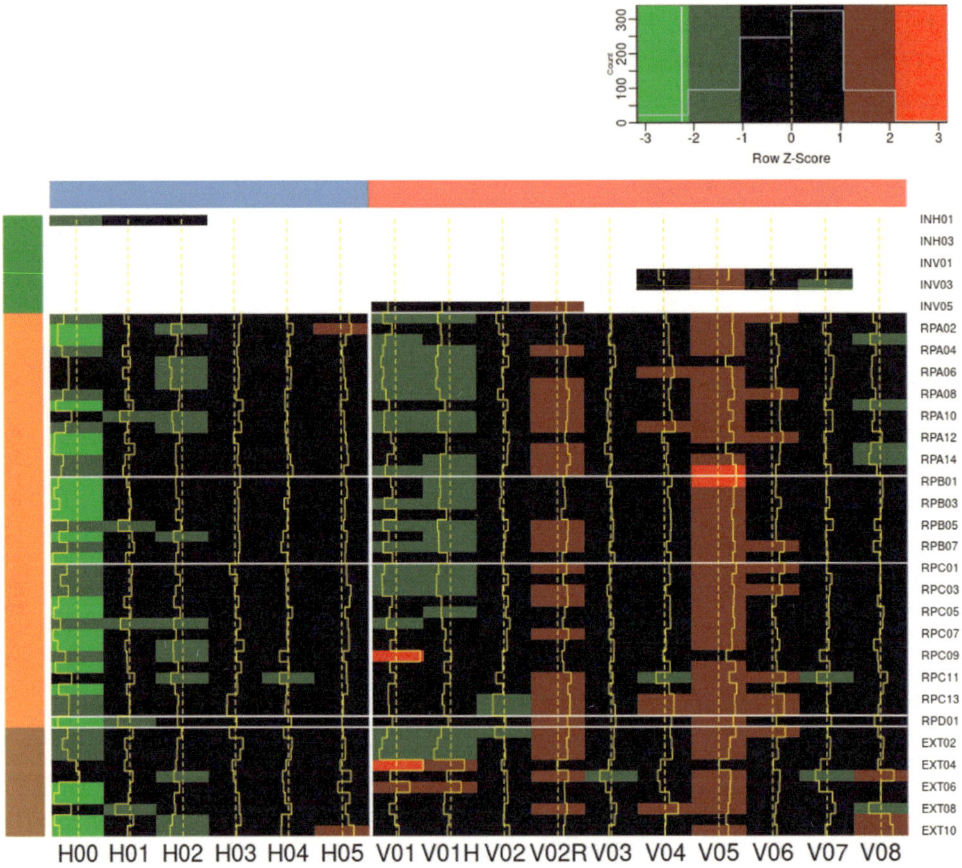

Figure 4.
*Target (columns) and ligand (rows) complex docking results. Heatmap of binding free-energy change estimates, using a color-based code according to the Z-score value through row analysis. Targets are grouped as host proteins (blue) and virus proteins (pink). Ligands are grouped by control set (green), potential repurposing drugs (orange), and others (brown). IDs correspond to those defined in **Tables 1–3**. Black shades represent ligands around the set's mean. In green shades, ligands with at least one negative standard deviation from the mean. Red shades represent ligands with at least one positive standard deviation from the mean.*

spike-ACE2 PPI [90]. In our study, saquinavir showed the best energy scores against TMPRSS2, ACE2, and the NSP8-NSP12 interface of the Rdrp complex, as shown in **Figure 5**. The transmembrane serine protease 2 (TMPRRS2) is essential in several viral infections. Previous reports have shown that the inhibition of this target significantly reduces SARS-CoV-2 entry in lung cells at nM concentrations and therefore the viral infection [91]. Saquinavir also presented the best energy scores against the ACE2 active site, a critical host target needed to initiate entry through the formation of the spike-ACE2 quaternary complex. In this scenario, conformational changes upon ligand binding into the catalytic cavity may shift the relative positions of the receptor's interface residues that bind to the spike protein and prevent the anchoring of the spike on host cells [92]. However, because saquinavir targets the catalytic site of ACE2, the main activity of this enzyme in the renin-angiotensin system requires further investigation of its biological effect as a competitive inhibitor [93]. In addition, our results show that this drug targets the Rdrp replication complex, which is consistent with the previous results reported in the literature [55, 94]. Interestingly, saquinavir appears to

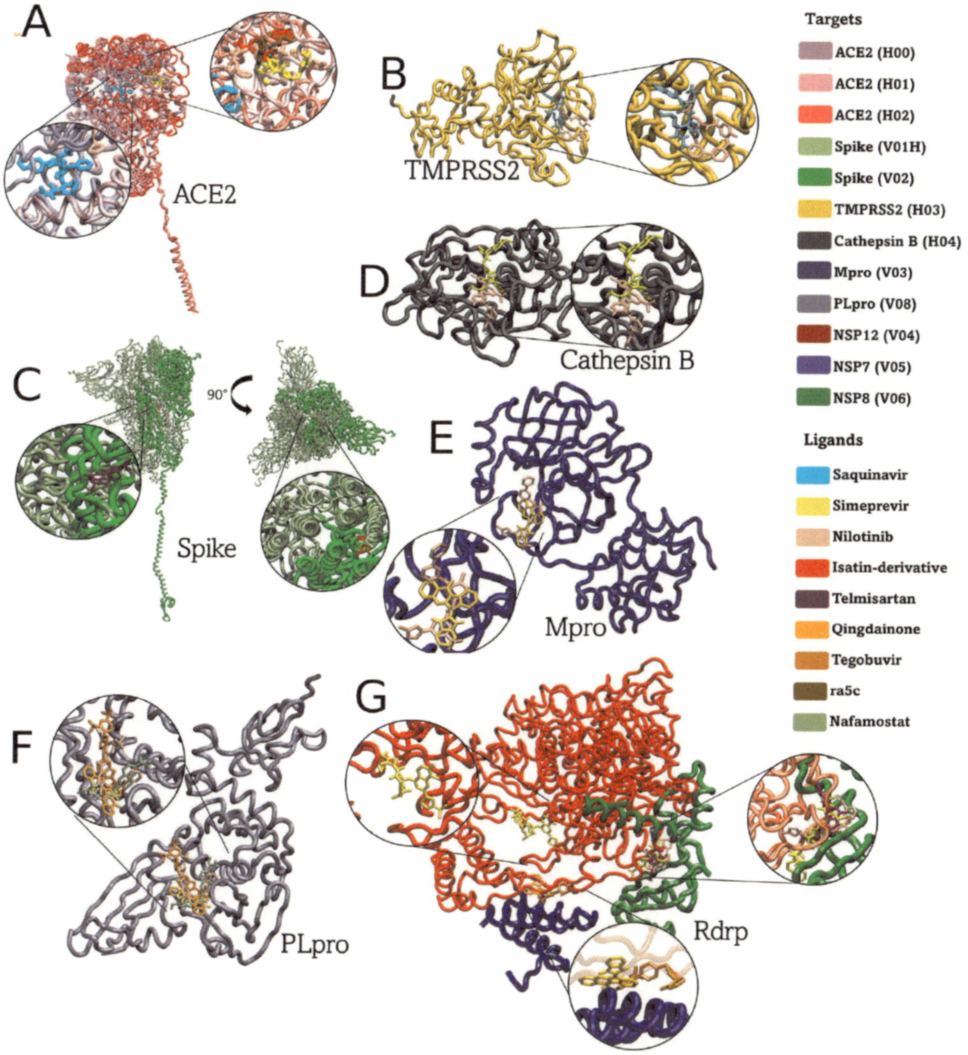

Figure 5.
Target-ligand complex conformations of potential drugs for repurposing. Molecular docking against viral and host targets relevant in the SARS-CoV-2 infection cycle. A. Superposition of ACE2 target (H00, H01, and H02) docked with saquinavir (cyan), isatin-derivative (red), nilotinib (pink), rac5c (brown), and simeprevir (yellow). B. TMPRSS2 docked with saquinavir (cyan) and nilotinib (pink). C. Spike docked with telmisartan (purple) and isatin-derivative (red). D. Cathepsin B docked with nilotinib and simeprevir (yellow). E. Mpro docked with nilotinib (pink) and qingdainone (orange). F. PLpro docked with nafamostat (green), nilotinib (pink), qingdainone (orange), and tegobuvir (dark orange). G. Superposition of NSP12 and NSP7 and NSP8 cofactors docked with simeprevir (yellow), tegobuvir (dark orange), nilotinib (pink), telmisartan (purple), qingdainone (orange), and saquinavir (cyan), created with the visual molecular dynamics (VMD) [84].

target two essential steps, compromising the entry and viral replication of the SARS-CoV-2.

On the other hand, simeprevir also showed the best energy scores on targets relevant to viral entry and replication, including the active cavities of ACE2, cathepsin B, NSP12, and the Rdrp complex interface. We show a molecular visualization of these results in panels A, C, and G of **Figure 5**. This drug is a protease inhibitor that has presented potent *in vitro* suppression of SARS-CoV-2 replication at μ M range in Vero

E6 cell lines [95]. It is a macrocyclic drug that forms a non-covalent bond within the active site of the hepatitis C virus (HCV) NS3/4A protease, which has a similar three-dimensional arrangement to SARS-CoV-2 Mpro catalytic residues [96]. Simeprevir binds to ACE2 in a quaternary complex inhibition mechanism, analogous to saquinavir, concomitant with the reported disruption of spike-ACE2 PPI [90]. However, the binding does not occur directly at the active site as saquinavir but in the same but larger cavity. Additionally, this drug targets the peptidase activity of cathepsin B, which is a crucial step in spike activation and viral entry. ACE2 was previously proposed as a strategic target to limit viral infection by targeting the cathepsin-mediated entry pathway, decreasing the viral infection efficiency [15, 97]. Simeprevir also showed the best results for the Rdrp complex. Consistent with our results, biochemical assays show low Rdrp replication efficiency after treatment with this drug [95].

5.2 Nilotinib targeting viral entry, polyprotein processing, and Rdrp quaternary complex

Nilotinib is used to treat chronic myelogenous leukemia as a Bcr-Abl tyrosine kinase antagonist. Our results suggest the potential inhibition of six targets involved in the SARS-CoV-2 infection process, including the catalytic cavities of enzyme targets ACE2, TMPRSS2, cathepsin B, Mpro, and the PLpro-ISG15 and Rdrp's NSP8-NSP12 interfaces. We show a molecular visualization of these results in **Figure 5**. Reports suggest that nilotinib can inhibit the SARS-CoV and SARS-CoV-2 infection processes, but not MERS-CoV. Interestingly, the latter does not use ACE2 as a cell receptor [98, 99]. This observation is particularly interesting since other reports suggest that nilotinib can destabilize the SARS-CoV-2 spike-ACE2 complex [54]. According to our results, nilotinib might prevent the spike priming and activation since it showed the best energy scores against TMPRSS2 and cathepsin B at the active site cavities. These findings represent a potential inhibition of two independent priming pathways. Moreover, nilotinib potentially inhibits the Mpro and Rdrp complex and is consistent with previous *in vitro* and *in silico* results [55, 100].

Interestingly, nilotinib also had the best energy scores against PLpro. In addition to PLpro's essential protease activity in the processing of pp1a polyprotein, it is also implicated in host immune innate response evasion mechanisms as described in Section 4.4. The inhibition of PLpro decreases the exacerbated immune response, as described by other members of the Bcr-Abl inhibitors family, for example, ponatinib, which protects against cytokine storm in mouse models [101, 102].

5.3 An isatin-derivative and telmisartan targeting SARS-CoV-2 entry

Isatin-derivatives have shown potential antiviral properties, some of them with promising results against HCV, SARS-CoV [103, 104], and SARS-CoV-2 [46]. In particular, the compound 1-(naphthalen-2-ylmethyl)-2,3-dioxoindoline-5-carboxamide inhibits Mpro from SARS-CoV-2. Therefore, we decided to evaluate it against our whole set of targets. It presented the best score against the ACE2 active site, which might disrupt the spike-ACE2 interaction as discussed previously (see Section 5.1). Moreover, it also showed the best energy scores against the spike protein, precisely in the quaternary interface region of the homotrimer complex, and thus a plausible termination of the viral cycle at an early stage in the replication process.

Telmisartan is an anti-antihypertensive. There is evidence of a morbidity and mortality reduction in hospitalized patients infected with SARS-CoV-2 treated with this drug [105]. Telmisartan showed the best energy scores against a spike's cavity in the homotrimer quaternary interface. Therefore, the isatin-derivative could inhibit two targets involved in the viral entry (spike and ACE2), while telmisartan might prevent the spike homotrimer formation and the Rdrp complex. We show the molecular visualization of these results in panels A, C, and G of **Figure 5**.

5.4 Tegobuvir, qingdainone, and nafamostat targeting quaternary interface regions

Tegobuvir is a non-nucleoside inhibitor of the NS5B polymerase of HCV. Our results suggest that this drug may prevent the formation of the Rdrp quaternary complex. Previously, *in silico* results reported tegobuvir as a potential inhibitor of Rdrp active site [106]. According to our data, tegobuvir did not achieve the selection criteria at the Rdrp active site. However, it shows a negative Z-score value at the NSP7-NSP12 interface region, which may compromise the RNA synthesis efficiency of the complex since its importance along with NSP8 for the Rdrp enzymatic activity [107]. Moreover, tegobuvir, nafamostat, and qingdainone presented the best binding free-energy change estimates on a cavity of PLpro in the vicinity of the interface of this target with ISG15, compromising an adequate immune response. In this manner, these drugs could avoid the formation of PLpro-ISG15 and the Rdrp quaternary complexes.

In addition, qingdainone also showed the potential inhibitory activity on Mpro active site, suggesting that this drug might completely disrupt the polyprotein processing stage by targeting both proteases, Mpro and PLpro. We show a molecular visualization of these results in **Figure 5**.

5.5 Nafamostat and rac5c as potential inhibitors of PLpro and ACE2

We included nafamostat and rac5c in our ligand sets due to evidence suggesting their inhibitory capacity against TMPRSS2 [108] and PLpro [19], respectively. Neither ligand achieved the selection criteria for their expected targets despite being on the borderline with scores of −8.3 and − 9.3 kcal/mol, which indicates the selection criteria's exhaustiveness. However, nafamostat does achieve the best scores against PLpro's USP domain, while rac5c presented the best score on the ACE2 active site. We show these results in panels A and F of **Figure 5**.

6. Conclusions

We have theoretically identified nine drugs or compounds for potential drug repurposing against SARS-CoV-2 through a cavity-based blind molecular docking protocol (**Figure 6**). Interestingly, seven of them present potential inhibitory activity on multiple targets at different stages of the viral infection cycle, including innate immune evasion. We have implemented an in-house high-throughput virtual screening pipeline that successfully reproduces experimental data and findings from previous works. After the target's cavity detection and ranking by surface area, we used the pipeline to perform the numerous independent blind molecular docking rounds to achieve a sufficiently extensive conformational target-ligand complex search.

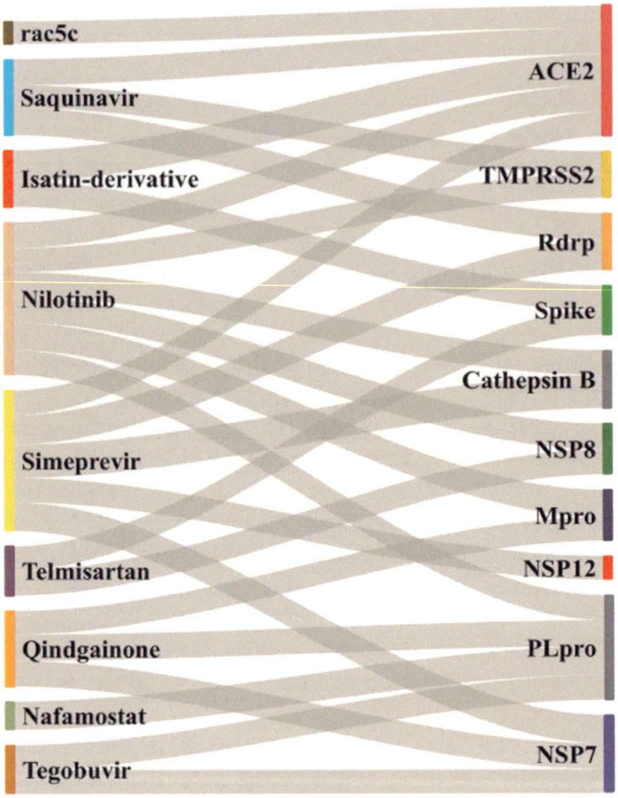

Figure 6.
Repurposing drugs (left) with corresponding potential inhibitory activity on multiple viral or host targets (right).

Experimental design is a critical step in every scientific study, for example, method validation by including a control group. Nonetheless, one has to be wary of the limitations of the methodology employed. In this case, molecular docking can be a good estimator for the most energetically favorable $T - L$ complex. However, the method does not explicitly consider solvent or thermodynamic parameters. Hence, molecular docking results should be taken as the input of other methodologies to further the study, for example, molecular dynamics.

We analyzed the molecular binding predictions through rigorous visualization and Z-score-based statistical algorithms to identify the potential drugs for repurposing. In this context, our findings suggest that:

- Saquinavir and simeprevir could target viral entry and Rdrp complex quaternary formation,
- Nilotinib could target viral entry, polyprotein processing, and Rdrp quaternary complex formation,
- An isatin-derivative and telmisartan could target SARS-CoV-2 entry into the host,
- Tegobuvir, qingdainone, and nafamostat could target quaternary interface Rdrp regions, and

- Nafamostat and rac5c could be potential inhibitors of PLpro and ACE2.

These results are relevant in understanding the SARS-CoV-2 drug's molecular mechanisms and further clinical treatment development, either at a single or multi-target activity.

Acknowledgements

The authors acknowledge funding from the Consejo Nacional de Ciencia y Tecnología México [grant number 132376] and Fondo Sectorial de Investigación para la Educación [grant number A1-S-17041] to MCT. All computations and analyses reported here were performed at the bmdhpc computing resources of the Biomolecular Diversity Lab (tripplab.com) at CINVESTAV Unidad Monterrey, México.

Conflict of interest

The authors declare no conflict of interest. The funders had no role in the design of the study; in the collection, analyses, or interpretation of data; in the writing of the manuscript, or in the decision to publish the results.

Abbreviations

ACE2	Angiotensin-converting enzyme 2
COVID-19	Coronavirus disease 19
HCV	Hepatitis C Virus
HTVS	High-throughput virtual screening
ISG15	Interferon-stimulated gene 15
MERS-CoV	Middle East respiratory syndrome coronavirus
Mpro	Main protease
PLpro	Papain-like protease
PPI	Protein-protein interactions
RBD	Receptor binding domain
Rdrp complex	RNA-dependent RNA polymerase complex
SARS-CoV	Severe acute respiratory syndrome coronavirus
SARS-CoV-2	Severe acute respiratory syndrome coronavirus 2
ssRNA	Single-stranded ribonucleic acid
TMPRSS2	Transmembrane serine protease 2

Appendix A

Li-Ta	H00	H01	H02	H03	H04	H05	V01	V01H	V02	V02R	V03	V04	V05	V06	V07	V08
INH01	−9.5	−7.3	−7.7													
INH02				−6												
INH03					−6.2											
INH04						−9										
INV01											−7.2					
INV02												−7.5	−5.5	−6.7	−7.8	
INV03												−7.6	−5.7	−6.6	−8.6	
INV04																−9.8
INV05							−6	−6	−4.1	−3.4						

Table A-1.
VINA scores of the conformation with the lowest scores after 30 independent cycles of each target–ligand pair for the enzymatic known inhibitors included.

Li-Ta	H00	H01	H02	H03	H04	H05	V01	V01H	V02	V02R	V03	V04	V05	V06	V07	V08
RPA01	−9.8	−8.5	−7.9	−6.8	−8	−6.6	−9.7	−9.6	−8.9	−6.8	−7.7	−7.5	−5.6	−6.5	−7.1	−8.8
RPA02	−11.4	−8.8	−10.3	−8.2	−8.1	−7.5	−9.3	−10	−9.4	−7.7	−8.7	−8.2	−6.9	−8.8	−9.2	−9.2
RPA03	−8.6	−6.5	−6.9	−5.9	−6.3	−5.9	−7.6	−7.3	−5.9	−5.7	−6.6	−5.9	−4.7	−5.9	−5.9	−7.5
RPA04	−9.8	−8.7	−8.7	−7.6	−7.6	−7.8	−9.5	−9.4	−7.8	−6.6	−7.4	−7.3	−6	−7	−7.6	−8.4
RPA05	−6.1	−5	−6.6	−4.8	−5.3	−4.9	−6.8	−6.7	−4.6	−4.2	−4.6	−4.2	−4.3	−4.5	−4.3	−6
RPA06	−7.3	−7	−7.6	−5.7	−5.8	−5.9	−7.8	−7.8	−6.4	−5.2	−6.1	−5	−4.5	−5.8	−5.3	−7.3
RPA07	−7.3	−6.4	−7.7	−5.9	−6	−5.9	−7.9	−7.9	−6.4	−5.3	−6.3	−5.6	−4.7	−5.9	−5.7	−7.2
RPA08	−9.5	−8	−7.9	−7.3	−7.9	−6.7	−8.9	−8.9	−8.3	−5.9	−8.2	−6.9	−5.3	−6.2	−6.9	−8.1
RPA09	−8.9	−6.3	−7.1	−5.9	−7	−6.8	−7.4	−7.2	−6.3	−5.7	−7	−6.2	−5.7	−5.9	−6.9	−7.7
RPA10	−4.7	−5	−5.1	−3.9	−4.3	−4	−5.2	−5.2	−4.1	−3.4	−4.5	−3.6	−3	−3.6	−3.7	−4.7
RPA11	−7.8	−6.6	−7.5	−5.6	−6.7	−6	−7.8	−7.8	−6.2	−5.3	−6.6	−5.1	−5.1	−5.4	−5.6	−7.3
RPA12	−11.6	−9.1	−8.9	−8.7	−8.8	−8	−9.2	−9	−7.8	−7.5	−8.9	−8.9	−6.5	−7.1	−8.8	−8.3
RPA13	−12	−7.7	−9.5	−8	−8.5	−7.7	−8.8	−9.1	−7.9	−7	−9.4	−8	−7.4	−7.3	−8.6	−9.9
RPA14	−10.5	−9.2	−9.5	−8.3	−8.3	−7.8	−9.8	−9.9	−8.2	−7	−8.5	−8.4	−6.8	−7.7	−8.9	−10.1
RPA15	−10.9	−9.4	−9.3	−7.8	−7.8	−8.2	−10.1	−9.9	−8.7	−7.2	−8.7	−8	−6	−8	−7.9	−9
RPB01	−11.1	−8.7	−9.3	−7.6	−8.3	−7.7	−9.1	−9.8	−8.8	−7.5	−8.9	−7.3	−5.8	−7.8	−8.3	−8
RPB02	−11.3	−7.8	−8.8	−7.5	−7.7	−7.1	−8.4	−9.3	−8.2	−6.8	−7.7	−7.4	−5.7	−7.4	−7.9	−7.5
RPB03	−10.6	−7.8	−8.5	−7.5	−8.6	−7.6	−9.7	−9.6	−8.6	−6.9	−8	−7.3	−5.9	−6.8	−7.6	−7.8
RPB04	−11.8	−8	−9	−7.6	−8.1	−7.6	−8	−8.6	−8.2	−7.5	−7.9	−7.2	−6.2	−7.4	−8.2	−8
RPB05	−10.4	−10.7	−9	−8.2	−8.9	−8.4	−11	−10.9	−8	−6.9	−8.3	−7.6	−6.2	−8.1	−7.6	−9.7
RPB06	−10.7	−7.7	−9.4	−7.5	−8.8	−7.4	−9.1	−9.7	−7.9	−6.7	−7.8	−7.3	−6.1	−7.6	−8.2	−8
RPB07	−8	−6.3	−7.3	−6.3	−7.6	−6.4	−8.3	−8.1	−6.8	−5.8	−7	−6.6	−5	−5.5	−6.8	−7.6
RPB08	−11.6	−8.6	−9	−7.6	−8.2	−7.6	−8.6	−8.5	−8.4	−7.4	−7.6	−7.2	−6.1	−7.1	−7.9	−8.2

Li-Ta	H00	H01	H02	H03	H04	H05	V01	V01H	V02	V02R	V03	V04	V05	V06	V07	V08
RPC01	−7.6	−6.1	−7.2	−7	−6.7	−5.9	−7.7	−7.7	−6.5	−5.4	−6.6	−5.9	−4.5	−5.1	−6.4	−6.4
RPC02	−10.3	−7.7	−8.3	−7.7	−8.2	−7.3	−9.9	−9.8	−7.4	−7.2	−8.1	−7.2	−6.1	−7	−7.3	−8
RPC03	−8.1	−6.7	−7.8	−7	−7.2	−5.9	−8.6	−8.6	−7.1	−5.8	−7.4	−6.8	−5.1	−5.8	−6.6	−6.9
RPC04	−12.3	−10.2	−10.7	−8.9	−9.6	−8.3	−10	−10.7	−8.8	−7.9	−9.7	−8.6	−7.2	−8.9	−9.1	−9.8
RPC05	−12.9	−8.7	−9.3	−8.8	−8.2	−8.4	−10	−10.4	−8.6	−7.7	−9.1	−8	−6.5	−9	−8.6	−8.4
RPC06	−11	−9.8	−9.8	−7.7	−8.6	−7.6	−9.9	−9.6	−7.6	−7.7	−8.1	−7.6	−6.2	−8	−8.1	−8.1
RPC07	−12.5	−8.9	−9.8	−8.6	−9	−7.8	−8.9	−9.5	−8.4	−7.2	−9.1	−8.7	−6.9	−8.1	−8.8	−8.9
RPC08	−11.5	−9.5	−10.2	−7.9	−9	−8.1	−9.7	−9.7	−8.6	−8.1	−8.6	−8.8	−7.3	−8.1	−8.7	−9.8
RPC09	−10.9	−9.3	−10.4	−8.6	−10.3	−8.6	−4.9	−8.7	−9.1	−8.1	−8.4	−9.1	−7.6	−8.3	−10	−9.3
RPC10	−11.2	−8.7	−9	−7.7	−8.4	−7.9	−9.2	−9.2	−8.6	−7.7	−8.6	−7.8	−6.4	−7.9	−8.1	−8.7
RPC11	−8.5	−7.4	−9.1	−7.7	−8.8	−7.4	−8	−7.9	−8.7	−6.5	−7.7	−8.8	−6.8	−6.6	−8.9	−7.2
RPC12	−10.3	−8.3	−8.9	−7.7	−8.1	−7.3	−8.9	−8.7	−8.1	−6.7	−8.2	−7.4	−5.8	−7.6	−7.5	−7.6
RPC13	−6.3	−5.5	−5.9	−6.2	−5.7	−5.4	−6.2	−6.2	−6.5	−4.4	−5.3	−4.7	−4.1	−4.5	−5.5	−5.5
RPC14	−6.4	−5.5	−6	−6.3	−5.8	−5.4	−6.2	−6.1	−6.6	−4.3	−5.1	−4.6	−3.9	−4.4	−5.4	−5.7
RPD01	−11	−9.9	−9	−8.1	−7.9	−8.3	−8.8	−8.6	−8.1	−7	−7.7	−7.4	−6.4	−7.8	−7.7	−9.1
EXT01	−6.3	−5.1	−5.5	−5.9	−5.8	−5.3	−6.2	−6.2	−6.2	−4.4	−5.1	−4.9	−3.9	−4.3	−5.3	−5.6
EXT02	−10	−8.4	−8.5	−6.5	−7.1	−7.2	−9.8	−9.6	−7.6	−6.3	−7.3	−6.6	−6	−7	−7.1	−7.2
EXT03	−9	−7.8	−8.3	−6.5	−6.9	−6.8	−10.1	−10	−7.1	−5.7	−6.8	−6.1	−5.7	−6.4	−6.8	−6.9
EXT04	−8	−9	−9.6	−8.4	−8.2	−7.9	0.9	−3.1	−8.2	−7.5	−8.2	−8.7	−7.2	−7.2	−9.3	−8.2
EXT05	−6.2	−6.1	−7.2	−6.5	−6.9	−5.6	−6.9	−6.7	−6.1	−5.4	−7.4	−7	−5.3	−5.7	−7.4	−5.2
EXT06	−9.6	−6.9	−7.4	−6.9	−7.6	−7.5	−5.1	−5.5	−6.5	−6	−7.7	−7.6	−5.4	−6	−8	−6.9
EXT07	−9.9	−7.3	−8.1	−6.7	−7.5	−6.3	−7.2	−7.8	−6.7	−6.3	−7.2	−6.6	−5.9	−6.5	−6.5	−7.1
EXT08	−6	−6.8	−6.1	−4.9	−5	−5	−6	−6	−5.3	−4.4	−4.8	−4	−4.4	−5	−4.5	−6.5

Li-Ta	H00	H01	H02	H03	H04	H05	V01	V01H	V02	V02R	V03	V04	V05	V06	V07	V08
EXT09	−11.2	−7	−9.2	−6.7	−8.6	−6.6	−7.8	−7.8	−7.6	−6.4	−7	−7.4	−6.4	−7.2	−7	−6.1
EXT10	−9.7	−7.7	−9	−7.3	−8.3	−6.1	−7.1	−7.8	−6.8	−6.7	−7.7	−7.4	−6.3	−6.9	−7.6	−6

Table A-2.
VINA scores of the conformation with the lowest scores after 30 independent cycles of each target–ligand pair for the set of ligands evaluated.

Author details

Aldo Herrera-Rodulfo, Mariana Andrade-Medina and Mauricio Carrillo-Tripp*
Biomolecular Diversity Laboratory, Centro de Investigación y de Estudios Avanzados del IPN Unidad Monterrey, Apodaca, Nuevo León, México

*Address all correspondence to: mauricio.carrillo@cinvestav.mx

References

[1] Costa V, Moreli M, Saivish M. The emergence of SARS, MERS and novel SARS-2 coronaviruses in the 21st century. Archives of Virology. 2020;**165**: 1517-1526

[2] WHO. Severe Acute Respiratory Syndrome. SARS. Available from: https://www.emro.who.int/health-topics/severe-acute-respiratory-syndrome/introduction.html

[3] WHO. Middle East Respiratory Syndrome. MERS Situation Update. Available from: https://www.emro.who.int/health-topics/mers-cov/mers-outbreaks.html

[4] World-Health-Organization WHO Coronavirus (COVID-19) Dashboard. Available from: https://covid19.who.int

[5] Ye Z, Yuan S, Yuen K, Fung S, Chan C, Jin D. Zoonotic origins of human coronaviruses. International Journal of Biological Sciences. 2020;**16**: 1686-1697

[6] Elezkurtaj S, Greuel S, Ihlow J, Michaelis E, Bischoff P, Kunze C, et al. Causes of death and comorbidities in hospitalized patients with COVID-19. Scientific Reports. 2021;**11**(1):4263

[7] Lubin J, Zardecki C, Dolan E, Lu C, Shen Z, Dutta S, et al. Evolution of the SARS-CoVscp-2 proteome in three dimensions (3D) during the first 6 months of the COVIDscp-19 pandemic. Proteins. Structure, Function, and Bioinformatics. 2021;**90**:1054-1080

[8] Liu Y, Grimm M, Wen-Dai M-H, Xiao Z, Cao Y. CB-Dock: A web server for cavity detection-guided protein–ligand blind docking. Acta Pharmacologica Sinica. 2019;**41**:138-144

[9] Liang J, Woodward C, Edelsbrunner H. Anatomy of protein pockets and cavities: Measurement of binding site geometry and implications for ligand design. Protein Science. 1998;**7**: 1884-1897

[10] Bienstock R. Computational drug design targeting protein-protein interactions. Current Pharmaceutical Design. 2012;**18**:1240-1254

[11] Chung-Chang, Lin S, Satange R, Lin S, Sun S, Wu H, et al. Targeting protein-protein interaction interfaces in COVID-19 drug discovery. Computational and Structural Biotechnology Journal. 2021; **19**:2246-2255

[12] Cha Y, Erez T, Reynolds I, Kumar D, Ross J, Koytiger G, et al. Drug repurposing from the perspective of pharmaceutical companies. British Journal of Pharmacology. 2017;**175**: 168-180

[13] Pushpakom S, Iorio F, Eyers P, Escott K, Hopper S, Wells A, et al. Drug repurposing: Progress, challenges and recommendations. Nature Reviews Drug Discovery. 2018;**18**:41-58

[14] Xiu S, Dick A, Ju H, Mirzaie S, Abdi F, Cocklin S, et al. Inhibitors of SARS-CoV-2 Entry: Current and future opportunities. Journal of Medicinal Chemistry. 2020;**63**:12256-12274

[15] Padmanabhan P, Desikan R, Dixit N. Targeting TMPRSS2 and cathepsin B/L together may be synergistic against SARS-CoV-2 infection. PLOS Computational Biology. 2020;**16**: e1008461

[16] Arya R, Kumari S, Pandey B, Mistry H, Bihani S, Das A, et al.

Structural insights into SARS-CoV-2 proteins. Journal of Molecular Biology. 2021;**433**:166725

[17] Beyer D, Forero A. Mechanisms of antiviral immune evasion of SARS-CoV-2. Journal of Molecular Biology. 2021;**434**(6):167265

[18] Liu G, Lee J, Parker Z, Acharya D, Chiang J, Gent M, et al. ISG15-dependent activation of the sensor MDA5 is antagonized by the SARS-CoV-2 papain-like protease to evade host innate immunity. Nature Microbiology. 2021;**6**: 467-478

[19] Klemm T, Ebert G, Calleja D, Allison C, Richardson L, Bernardini J, et al. Mechanism and Inhibition of SARS-CoV-2 PLpro. Cold Spring Harbor Laboratory; 2020

[20] Ma C, Sacco MD, Xia Z, Lambrinidis G, Townsend JA, Hu Y, et al. Discovery of SARS-CoV-2 Papain-like Protease Inhibitors through a Combination of High-Throughput Screening and a FlipGFP-Based Reporter Assay. ACS Central Science. 2021;**7**(7):1245-1260

[21] Pettersen E, Goddard T, Huang C, Couch G, Greenblatt D, Meng E, et al. UCSF Chimera?A visualization system for exploratory research and analysis. Journal of Computational Chemistry. 2004;**25**:1605-1612

[22] Morris G, Huey R, Lindstrom W, Sanner M, Belew R, Goodsell D, et al. AutoDock4 and AutoDockTools4: Automated docking with selective receptor flexibility. Journal of Computational Chemistry. 2009;**30**: 2785-2791

[23] Gurwitz D. Angiotensin receptor blockers as tentative SARS-CoV-2 therapeutics. Drug Development Research. 2020;**81**:537-540

[24] Nejat R, Sadr A, Freitas B, Crabttree J, Pegan S, Tripp R, et al. Losartan inhibits SARS-CoV-2 replication in vitro. Journal of Pharmacy & Pharmaceutical Sciences. 2021;**24**:390-399

[25] Rothlin R, Vetulli H, Duarte M, Pelorosso F. Telmisartan as tentative angiotensin receptor blocker therapeutic for COVID -19. Drug Development Research. 2020;**81**:768-770

[26] McKee D, Sternberg A, Stange U, Laufer S, Naujokat C. Candidate drugs against SARS-CoV-2 and COVID-19. Pharmacological Research. 2020;**157**: 104859

[27] Vankadari N. Arbidol: A potential antiviral drug for the treatment of SARS-CoV-2 by blocking trimerization of the spike glycoprotein. International Journal of Antimicrobial Agents. 2020; **56**:105998

[28] Breining P, Fralund A, Hajen J, Gunst J, Staerke N, Saedder E, et al. Camostat mesylate against SARS-CoV-2 and COVID-19—Rationale, dosing and safety. Basic & Clinical Pharmacology & Toxicology. 2020;**128**:204-212

[29] Halder UC. Predicted antiviral drugs Darunavir, Amprenavir, Rimantadine and Saquinavir can potentially bind to neutralize SARS-CoV-2 conserved proteins. Journal of Biological Research-Thessaloniki. 2021;**28**(1):18

[30] Braz H, Moraes Silveira J, Marinho A, Moraes M, Moraes Filho M, Monteiro H, et al. In silico study of azithromycin, chloroquine and hydroxychloroquine and their potential mechanisms of action against SARS-CoV-2 infection. International Journal of Antimicrobial Agents. 2020;**56**:106119

[31] COVID-19 update: Baricitinib (Olumiant) FDA-approved for

treatment of COVID-19. Medical Letter on Drugs and Therapeutics. 2022;**64**: 1652

[32] Jorgensen S, Tse C, Burry L, Dresser LB. A review of pharmacology, safety, and emerging clinical experience in COVID-19. Pharmacotherapy. The Journal of Human Pharmacology and Drug Therapy. 2020;**40**:843-856

[33] Yousefi H, Mashouri L, Okpechi S, Alahari N, Alahari S. Repurposing existing drugs for the treatment of COVID-19/SARS-CoV-2 infection: A review describing drug mechanisms of action. Biochemical Pharmacology. 2021; **183**:114296

[34] Parra-Medina R, Sarmiento-Monroy J, Rojas-Villarraga A, Garavito E, Montealegre-Gómez G, Gómez-López A. Colchicine as a possible therapeutic option in COVID-19 infection. Clinical Rheumatology. 2020;**39**:2485-2486

[35] Ma C, Hu Y, Townsend J, Lagarias P, Marty M, Kolocouris A, et al. Ebselen, Disulfiram, Carmofur, PX-12, Tideglusib, and Shikonin Are Nonspecific Promiscuous SARS-CoV-2 Main Protease Inhibitors. ACS Pharmacology and Translational Science. 2020;**3**(6):1265-1277

[36] Chen T, Fei C, Chen Y, Sargsyan K, Chang C, Yuan H, et al. Synergistic inhibition of SARS-CoV-2 replication using disulfiram/ebselen and remdesivir. ACS Pharmacology & Translational Science. 2021;**4**:898-907

[37] Haritha C, Sharun K, Jose B. Ebselen, a new candidate therapeutic against SARS-CoV-2. International Journal of Surgery. 2020;**84**:53-56

[38] Wu C, Liu Y, Yang Y, Zhang P, Zhong W, Wang Y, et al. Analysis of therapeutic targets for SARS-CoV-2 and discovery of potential drugs by computational methods. Acta Pharmaceutica Sinica B. 2020;**10**:766-788

[39] Junior A, Tolouei S, Reis Livero F, Gasparotto F, Boeing T, Souza P. Natural agents modulating ACE2: A review of compounds with potential against SARS-CoV-2 infections. Current Pharmaceutical Design. 2021;**27**: 1588-1596

[40] Vivek-Ananth R, Rana A, Rajan N, Biswal H, Samal A. In Silico identification of potential natural product inhibitors of human proteases key to SARS-CoV-2 infection. Molecules. 2020;**25**:3822

[41] Rangel H, Ortega J, Maksoud S, Pujol F, Serrano M. SARS-CoV-2 host tropism: An in silico analysis of the main cellular factors. Virus Research. 2020; **289**:198154

[42] Yamamoto M, Kiso M, Sakai-Tagawa Y, Iwatsuki-Horimoto K, Imai M, Takeda M, et al. The anticoagulant nafamostat potently inhibits SARS-CoV-2 S protein-mediated fusion in a cell fusion assay system and viral infection in vitro in a cell-type-dependent manner. Viruses. 2020;**12**:629

[43] Greenspan P, Clark K, Tommasi R, Cowen S, McQuire L, Farley D, et al. Identification of dipeptidyl nitriles as potent and selective inhibitors of cathepsin B through structure-based drug design. Journal of Medicinal Chemistry. 2001;**44**:4524-4534

[44] Dorward J, Gbinigie O, Cai T, Roberts N, Garrett N, Hayward G, et al. The protease inhibitor lopinavir, boosted with ritonavir, as treatment for COVID-19: A rapid review. Antiviral Therapy. 2021;**25**:365-376

[45] Kim E, Choi S, Park J, Kwon Y, Lee J, Kim Y, et al. Use of darunavir-cobicistat

as a treatment option for critically Ill patients with SARS-CoV-2 infection. Yonsei Medical Journal. 2020;**61**:826

[46] Liu P, Liu H, Sun Q, Liang H, Li C, Deng X, et al. Potent inhibitors of SARS-CoV-2 3C-like protease derived from N-substituted isatin compounds. European Journal Of Medicinal Chemistry. 2020;**206**:112702

[47] Xie X, Muruato A, Zhang X, Lokugamage K, Fontes-Garfias C, Zou J, et al. A nanoluciferase SARS-CoV-2 for rapid neutralization testing and screening of anti-infective drugs for COVID-19. Nature Communications. 2020;**12**(1):3984

[48] Liu C, Boland S, Scholle M, Bardiot D, Marchand A, Chaltin P, et al. Dual inhibition of SARS-CoV-2 and human rhinovirus with protease inhibitors in clinical development. Antiviral Research. 2021;**187**:105020

[49] Schiefer I, Tapadar S, Litosh V, Siklos M, Scism R, Wijewickrama G, et al. Design, synthesis, and optimization of novel epoxide incorporating peptidomimetics as selective calpain inhibitors. Journal of Medicinal Chemistry. 2013;**56**:6054-6068

[50] Griffin J. SARS-CoV and SARS-CoV-2 main protease residue interaction networks change when bound to inhibitor N3. Journal of Structural Biology. 2020;**211**:107575

[51] Khan S, Attar F, Bloukh S, Sharifi M, Nabi F, Bai Q, et al. A review on the interaction of nucleoside analogues with SARS-CoV-2 RNA dependent RNA polymerase. International Journal of Biological Macromolecules. 2021;**181**: 605-611

[52] Ju J, Li X, Kumar S, Jockusch S, Chien M, Tao C, et al. Nucleotide analogues as inhibitors of SARS-CoV-2 Polymerase, a Key Drug Target for COVID-19. Journal of Proteome Research. 2020;**19**(11):4690-4697

[53] Tian-Wei, Wang H, Xue-Wu, Lu Y, Sheng-Guan, Feng-Dong, et al. In silico screening of potential spike glycoprotein inhibitors of SARS-CoV-2 with drug repurposing strategy. Chinese Journal of Integrative Medicine. 2020;**26**:663-669

[54] Razizadeh M, Nikfar M, Liu Y. Small molecules to destabilize the ACE2-RBD complex: A molecular dynamics study for potential COVID-19 therapeutics. American Chemical Society (ACS). 2020

[55] Ruan Z, Liu C, Guo Y, He Z, Huang X, Jia X, et al. SARS-CoV-2 and SARS-CoV: Virtual screening of potential inhibitors targeting RNA-dependent RNA polymerase activity (NSP12). Journal of Medical Virology. 2020;**93**: 389-400

[56] Rossetti CA. High dose of ascorbic acid used in sars covid-19 treatment: Scientific and clinical support for its therapeutic implementation. Ars Pharmaceutica. 2020;**61**(2):145-148

[57] Santaolalla A, Beckmann K, Kibaru J, Josephs D, Hemelrijck M, Irshad S. Association between vitamin D and novel SARS-CoV-2 respiratory dysfunction – A scoping review of current evidence and its implication for COVID-19 pandemic. Frontiers in Physiology. 2020;**11**:564387

[58] Alam M, Czajkowsky D, Islam M, Rahman M. The role of vitamin D in reducing SARS-CoV-2 infection: An update. International Immunopharmacology. 2021;**97**:107686

[59] Kinobe R, Owens L. A systematic review of experimental evidence for antiviral effects of ivermectin and an in

silico analysis of ivermectin's possible mode of action against SARS-CoV-2. Fundamental & Clinical Pharmacology. 2021;**35**:260-276

[60] Venditto V, Haydar D, Abdel-Latif A, Gensel J, Anstead M, Pitts M, et al. Immunomodulatory effects of azithromycin revisited: Potential applications to COVID-19. Frontiers in Immunology. 2021;**12**:574425

[61] Mycroft-West C, Su D, Pagani I, Rudd T, Elli S, Gandhi N, et al. Heparin inhibits cellular invasion by SARS-CoV-2: Structural dependence of the interaction of the spike S1 receptor-binding domain with heparin. Thrombosis and Haemostasis. 2020; **120**:1700-1715

[62] Ye Z, Yuan S, Chan J, Zhang A, Yu C, Ong C, et al. Beneficial effect of combinational methylprednisolone and remdesivir in hamster model of SARS-CoV-2 infection. Emerging Microbes & Infections. High dose of ascorbic acid used in sars covid-19 treatment: scientific and clinical support for its therapeutic implementation. 2021: 291-304

[63] Javed H, Meeran M, Jha N, Ojha S. Carvacrol, a plant metabolite targeting viral protease (Mpro) and ACE2 in host cells can be a possible candidate for COVID-19. Frontiers in Plant Science. 2021;**11**:601335

[64] Romeo I, Mesiti F, Lupia A, Alcaro S. Current updates on naturally occurring compounds recognizing SARS-CoV-2 druggable targets. Molecules. 2021;**26**:632

[65] Berman H. The protein data bank. Nucleic Acids Research. 2000;**28**:235-242

[66] Jo S, Kim T, Iyer V, Im W. CHARMM-GUI: A web-based graphical user interface for CHARMM. Journal of Computational Chemistry. 2008;**29**: 1859-1865

[67] Towler P, Staker B, Prasad S, Menon S, Tang J, Parsons T, et al. ACE2 X-ray structures reveal a large hinge-bending motion important for inhibitor binding and catalysis. Journal of Biological Chemistry. 2004;**279**:17996-18007

[68] Yan R, Zhang Y, Li Y, Xia L, Guo Y, Zhou Q. Structural basis for the recognition of SARS-CoV-2 by full-length human ACE2. Science. 2020;**367**: 1444-1448

[69] Fraser B, Beldar S, Seitova A, Hutchinson A, Mannar D, Li Y, et al. Structure, Activity and Inhibition of Human TMPRSS2, A Protease Implicated in SARS-CoV-2 Activation. Cold Spring Harbor Laboratory; 2021

[70] Mirković B, Renko M, Turk S, Sosič I, Jevnikar Z, Obermajer N, et al. Novel mechanism of cathepsin inhibition by antibiotic nitroxoline and related compounds. ChemMedChem. 2011;**6**: 1351-1356

[71] Ljunggren A, Redzynia I, Alvarez-Fernandez M, Abrahamson M, Mort J, Krupa J, et al. Crystal structure of the parasite protease inhibitor chagasin in complex with a host target cysteine protease. Journal of Molecular Biology. 2007;**371**:137-153

[72] Woo H, Park S, Choi Y, Park T, Tanveer M, Cao Y, et al. Developing a fully glycosylated full-length SARS-CoV-2 spike protein model in a viral membrane. The Journal of Physical Chemistry B. 2020;**124**:7128-7137

[73] Walls A, Park Y, Tortorici M, Wall A, McGuire A, Veesler D. Structure, function, and antigenicity of the SARS-CoV-2 spike glycoprotein. Cell. 2020; **181**:281-292.e6

[74] Jin Z, Du X, Xu Y, Deng Y, Liu M, Zhao Y, et al. Structure of Mpro from SARS-CoV-2 and discovery of its inhibitors. Nature. 2020;**582**: 289-293

[75] Naydenova K, Muir K, Wu L, Zhang Z, Coscia F, Peet M, et al. Structure of the SARS-CoV-2 RNA-dependent RNA polymerase in the presence of favipiravir-RTP. Proceedings of The National Academy Of Sciences. 2021;**118**: e2021946118

[76] Gao Y, Yan L, Huang Y, Liu F, Zhao Y, Cao L, et al. Structure of the RNA-dependent RNA polymerase from COVID-19 virus. Science. 2020;**368**: 779-782

[77] Kirchdoerfer R, Ward A. Structure of the SARS-CoV nsp12 polymerase bound to nsp7 and nsp8 co-factors. Nature Communications. 2019;**10**(1):2342

[78] Ferreira L, Dos Santos R, Oliva G, Andricopulo A. Molecular docking and structure-based drug design strategies. Molecules. 2015;**20**:13384-13421

[79] Cao Y, Li L. Improved protein–ligand binding affinity prediction by using a curvature-dependent surface-area model. Bioinformatics. 2014;**30**: 1674-1680

[80] Zhao J, Cao Y, Zhang L. Exploring the computational methods for protein-ligand binding site prediction. Computational and Structural Biotechnology Journal. 2020;**18**: 417-426

[81] Trott O, Olson A. AutoDock Vina: Improving the speed and accuracy of docking with a new scoring function, efficient optimization, and multithreading. Journal of Computational Chemistry. 2009:**31**(2):455-461

[82] Yin W, Mao C, Luan X, Shen D, Shen Q, Su H, et al. Structural basis for inhibition of the RNA-dependent RNA polymerase from SARS-CoV-2 by remdesivir. Science. 2020;**368**:1499-1504

[83] Fink K, Nitsche A, Neumann M, Grossegesse M, Eisele K, Danysz W. Amantadine Inhibits SARS-CoV-2 In Vitro. Viruses. 2021;**13**:539

[84] Humphrey W, Dalke A, Schulten K. VMD – Visual molecular dynamics. Journal of Molecular Graphics. 1996;**14**: 33-38

[85] Cao X. ISG15 secretion exacerbates inflammation in SARS-CoV-2 infection. Nature Immunology. 2021;**22**:1360-1362

[86] Bello M, Martínez-Muñoz A, Balbuena-Rebolledo I. Identification of saquinavir as a potent inhibitor of dimeric SARS-CoV2 main protease through MM/GBSA. Journal of Molecular Modeling. 2020;**26**(12):340

[87] Raphael V, Shanmughan S. Computational evaluation of the inhibition efficacies of HIV antivirals on SARS-CoV-2 (COVID-19) protease and identification of 3D pharmacophore and hit compounds. Advances in Pharmacological and Pharmaceutical Sciences. 2020;**2020**:1-10

[88] Beck BR, Shin B, Choi Y, Park S, Kang K. Predicting commercially available antiviral drugs that may act on the novel coronavirus (SARS-CoV-2) through a drug-target interaction deep learning model. Computational and Structural Biotechnology Journal. 2020; **18**:784-790

[89] Mohamed K, Yazdanpanah N, Saghazadeh A, Rezaei N. Computational drug discovery and repurposing for the treatment of COVID-19: A systematic

review. Bioorganic Chemistry. 2021;**106**: 104490

[90] Brimacombe K, Zhao T, Eastman R, Hu X, Wang K, Backus M, et al. An OpenData portal to share COVID-19 Drug repurposing data in real time. bioRxiv [Preprint]. 2020

[91] Hoffmann M, Schroeder S, Kleine-Weber H, Müller M, Drosten C, Pöhlmann S. Nafamostat mesylate blocks activation of SARS-CoV-2: new treatment option for COVID-19. Antimicrobial Agents And Chemotherapy. 2020;**64**:e00754-e00720

[92] Teralı K, Baddal B, Gülcan H. Prioritizing potential ACE2 inhibitors in the COVID-19 pandemic: Insights from a molecular mechanics-assisted structure-based virtual screening experiment. Journal of Molecular Graphics and Modelling. 2020;**100**:107697

[93] Verdecchia P, Cavallini C, Spanevello A, Angeli F. The pivotal link between ACE2 deficiency and SARS-CoV-2 infection. European Journal of Internal Medicine. 2020;**76**: 14-20

[94] Alexpandi R, Mesquita J, Pandian S, Ravi A. Quinolines-based SARS-CoV-2 3CLpro and RdRp inhibitors and spike-RBD-ACE2 inhibitor for drug-repurposing against COVID-19: An in silico analysis. Frontiers in Microbiology. 2020;**11**:1796

[95] Lo H, Hui K, Lai H, He X, Khan K, Kaur S, et al. Simeprevir potently suppresses SARS-CoV-2 replication and synergizes with remdesivir. ACS Central Science. 2021;7:792-802

[96] Bafna K, Krug RM, Montelione GT. Structural Similarity of SARS-CoV2 Mpro and HCV NS3/4A Proteases Suggests New Approaches for Identifying Existing Drugs Useful as COVID-19 Therapeutics. ChemRxiv [Preprint]. 2020

[97] Hashimoto R, Sakamoto A, Deguchi S, Yi R, Sano E, Hotta A, et al. Dual inhibition of TMPRSS2 and Cathepsin Bprevents SARS-CoV-2 infection in iPS cells. Molecular Therapy - Nucleic Acids. 2021;**26**:1107-1114

[98] Cagno V, Magliocco G, Tapparel C, Daali Y. The tyrosine kinase inhibitor nilotinib inhibits SARS-CoV-2 in vitro. Basic & Clinical Pharmacology & Toxicology. 2020;**128**:621-624

[99] Dyall J, Coleman C, Hart B, Venkataraman T, Holbrook M, Kindrachuk J, et al. Repurposing of clinically developed drugs for treatment of middle east respiratory syndrome coronavirus infection. Antimicrobial Agents and Chemotherapy. 2014;**58**: 4885-4893

[100] Banerjee S, Yadav S, Banerjee S, Fakayode S, Parvathareddy J, Reichard W, et al. Drug repurposing to identify nilotinib as a potential SARS-CoV-2 main protease inhibitor: insights from a computational and in vitro study. Journal of Chemical Information And Modeling. 2021;**61**:5469-5483

[101] Mahmoudvand S, Shokri S. Interactions between SARS coronavirus 2 papain-like protease and immune system: A potential drug target for the treatment of COVID-19. Scandinavian Journal of Immunology. 2021;**94**(4): e13044

[102] Chen S, Liu G, Chen J, Hu A, Zhang L, Sun W, et al. Ponatinib protects mice from lethal influenza infection by suppressing cytokine storm. Frontiers in Immunology. 2019;**10**:1393

[103] Selvam P, Murgesh N, Chandramohan M, Clercq E, Keyaerts E, Vijgen L, et al. In vitro antiviral activity of some novel isatin derivatives against HCV and SARS-CoV viruses. Indian Journal of Pharmaceutical Sciences. 2008;**70**:91

[104] Zhou L, Liu Y, Zhang W, Wei P, Huang C, Pei J, et al. Isatin compounds as noncovalent SARS coronavirus 3C-like protease inhibitors. Journal of Medicinal Chemistry. 2006;**49**: 3440-3443

[105] Duarte M, Pelorosso F, Nicolosi L, Salgado M, Vetulli H, Aquieri A, et al. Telmisartan for treatment of Covid-19 patients: An open multicenter randomized clinical trial. EClinicalMedicine. 2021;**37**:100962

[106] Mosayebnia M, Bozorgi A, Rezaeianpour M, Kobarfard F. In silico prediction of SARS-CoV-2 main protease and polymerase inhibitors: 3D-Pharmacophore modelling. Journal of Biomolecular Structure and Dynamics. 2021:1-18

[107] Wang Q, Wu J, Wang H, Gao Y, Liu Q, Mu A, et al. Structural basis for RNA replication by the SARS-CoV-2 polymerase. Cell. 2020;**182**:417-428.e13

[108] Li K, Meyerholz D, Bartlett J, McCray P. The TMPRSS2 inhibitor nafamostat reduces SARS-CoV-2 pulmonary infection in mouse models of COVID-19. MBio. 2021;**12**(4):e0097021

Chapter 7

N1-(3-(Trifluoromethyl)Phenyl) Isophthalamide Derivatives as Promising Inhibitors of Vascular Endothelial Growth Factor Receptor: Pharmacophore-Based Design, Docking, and MM-PBSA/ MM-GBSA Binding Energy Estimation

Aliaksandr Faryna and Elena Kalinichenko

Abstract

Targeting protein kinases is a common approach for cancer treatment. In this study, a series of novel terephthalic and isophthalic derivatives were constructed as potential type 2 protein kinase inhibitors adapting pharmacophore features of approved anticancer drugs of this class. Inhibitory activity of designed structures was studied in silico against various cancer-related protein kinases and compared with that of known inhibitors. Obtained docking scores, MM-PBSA/MM-GBSA binding energy, and RF-Score-VS affinities suggest that N1-(3-(trifluoromethyl) phenyl) isophthalamide could be considered as promising scaffold for the development of novel protein kinase inhibitors which are able to target the inactive conformation of vascular endothelial growth factor receptor.

Keywords: terephthalic and isophthalic derivatives, anticancer activity, VEGFR, virtual screening, MM-PBSA/MM-GBSA, docking

1. Introduction

Since its approval in 2001, imatinib has revolutionized drug therapy of chronic myeloid leukemia (CML) [1, 2]. Imatinib is a selective inhibitor of a specific protein – BCR-ABL tyrosine kinase, which biosynthesis is encoded by the Philadelphia chromosome, which is characteristic for all CML cells [3, 4]. High and uncontrolled activity of this protein leads to disruption of cell signaling causing a rapid growth of the tumor tissue. Imatinib has secured more than 80% 8-year overall survival rate in patients with CML, almost double compared to the previous drugs generation [5, 6].

The clinical success of imatinib has fueled an explosion in the protein kinase inhibitor research. The strategy of blocking signaling pathways mediated by an overexpression or deregulation of certain protein kinases has proven to be effective in treating many other cancers as well as some non-cancer diseases. More than seventy drugs of this class have now been registered, targeting dozens of various kinase targets, which constitutes about 10% of the total number of kinases encoded by the human genome [7, 8]. Besides BCR-ABL, another large group of drugs targets various growth factors receptors (epidermal, platelet, vascular endothelial, etc.) [9, 10].

The use of protein kinase inhibitors for cancer treatment has some limitations. First of all, an important problem is drug resistance in patients. Resistance can occur initially (primary resistance) or over time (secondary resistance) [11–13]. One of the key mechanisms of secondary resistance is the emergence of the mutants of the primary target, which appears with the disease progression. Binding affinity of an inhibitor to the mutant target is significantly lower. In some cases, such mutations completely block binding [14–19].

The second key consideration is inhibitor selectivity. Since all protein kinases accept ATP as a substrate, there is a high structural similarity between the active sites of different protein kinases. An inhibitor usually does not act exclusively on its main target but can suppress, to some degree, the activity of some or many other kinase targets. So, such multitargetness can be a positive (e.g. when cancer cells express several types of kinases) or a negative factor – side inhibition can be the cause of adverse effects [20, 21]. Selectivity modulation becomes even more problematic with the disease progression as it is accompanied by further genetic degradation of cancer cells [22, 23]. For example, in the case of CML, the optimal choice for a second-line therapy inhibitor between dasatinib, bosutinib, and nilotinib can be made based on a personalized assessment of the actual kinase overexpression profile [24].

Since the efficacy of treatment with protein kinase inhibitors depends significantly on the time of treatment initiation, the most important property of a drug is its actual inhibitory activity, including that toward mutant targets. For example, nilotinib, a second-generation structural analog of imatinib, has been initially considered as a second-line therapy option [25]. Further investigations have showed that this drug could be more effective than imatinib as a first-line therapy being a more potent inhibitor of BCR-ABL and its mutants [26, 27].

Therefore, the search for the novel highly effective inhibitors of therapeutically relevant protein kinases with a given selectivity and the ability to suppress mutant targets is still an important scientific challenge.

In this context, the recent advances in the development of molecular modeling techniques for the search of biologically active compounds cannot be overlooked. The literature describes cases of successful application of pharmacophore screening [28, 29], molecular docking, and molecular dynamics [30–32] to identify new chemical structures with anti-kinase activity. In addition, the improvements in technical and theoretical background of machine learning algorithms have made it possible to adapt them, inter alia, for the modeling of protein-ligand interactions [33–36].

The present work continues our previous studies on the design of novel potential protein kinase inhibitors using directed pharmacophore design and molecular modeling [37, 38]. In this case, the object of such studies is new derivatives of terephthalic and isophthalic acids, which are designed in a manner to give the structures significant pharmacophore similarity to known type 2 protein kinase inhibitors.

The potential anti-kinase activity of the designed terephthalic and isophthalic acids derivatives has been investigated by molecular docking, molecular dynamics, as well as by using machine learning model for virtual screening RF-Score-VS [39].

2. Materials and methods

2.1 Design of target structures

X-ray diffraction data have revealed a number of common patterns in terms of binding of known protein kinase inhibitors to their targets. Two large groups of inhibitors can be distinguished. Type 1 inhibitors are direct ATP competitors and bind to the active center of the biologically active conformation of a protein kinase. Most of the approved inhibitors are type 1 inhibitors. However, in the case of imatinib, the binding is of a slightly different nature. The loop that links the two main lobes of BCR-ABL tyrosine kinase is flexible and in a certain position opens up an additional allosteric pocket adjacent immediately to the ATP binding site, thus extending the active center of the enzyme [40]. At the same time, the structure of the ATP pocket changes significantly, so it is unable to accept the natural substrate. Such inactive conformations can be seen for many others protein kinases. Inhibitors that bind to this inactive conformation of a protein kinase target are classified as type 2 inhibitors [41]. The described classification to this most common inhibitor classes is not perfectly strict, since there are stable intermediate kinase conformations with different volumes of allosteric pocket available and it is hard to classify ligand binding as type 1 or type 2 unambiguously [42].

In the structure of type 2 inhibitors, a number of key structural and pharmacophore features can be distinguished. Firstly, there is a benzamide fragment, most often with the 3-trifluoromethyl substituent in the benzene ring, which facilitates the formation of the necessary interactions, including hydrogen bonds, in the allosteric pocket of the active center. Secondly, the structure of type 2 inhibitors contains a heteroaromatic system, which in some sense imitates adenine but can form hydrogen bonds in the modified ATP pocket, which has been subjected to the structural changes upon the transition of a kinase to the inactive conformation. The relative orientation of these structural fragments is managed by the linker, which is usually represented by a benzene ring containing substituents in different positions [43–46].

In our previous studies, we have used the 4-methylbenzamide linker as a framework for constructing novel type 2 protein kinase inhibitors and that are allowed us to identify novel bioactive compounds with actual inhibitory activity against protein kinases [37, 38].

In this study, we have proposed that isophthalic and terephthalic acids transform into appropriate amides as a promising linkers for developing potential protein kinase inhibitors (**Figure 1**). In our opinion, the use of such linkers may be favorable for several reasons. For instance, these structures contain an amide bond, which is necessary for the formation of hydrogen bonds in the allosteric pocket of a kinase binding pocket. In addition, the overall size of linkers corresponds to those in the structures of known inhibitors. Moreover, the presence of a second carboxylic group may lead to the formation of hydrogen bonds in the ATP pocket. If compared to 4-methylbenzamide this linkers are more rigid, which may have a positive effect on kinase binding affinity. It is also important to note that we have used both isophthalic and terephthalic fragments to more fully study the conformational space of the linker

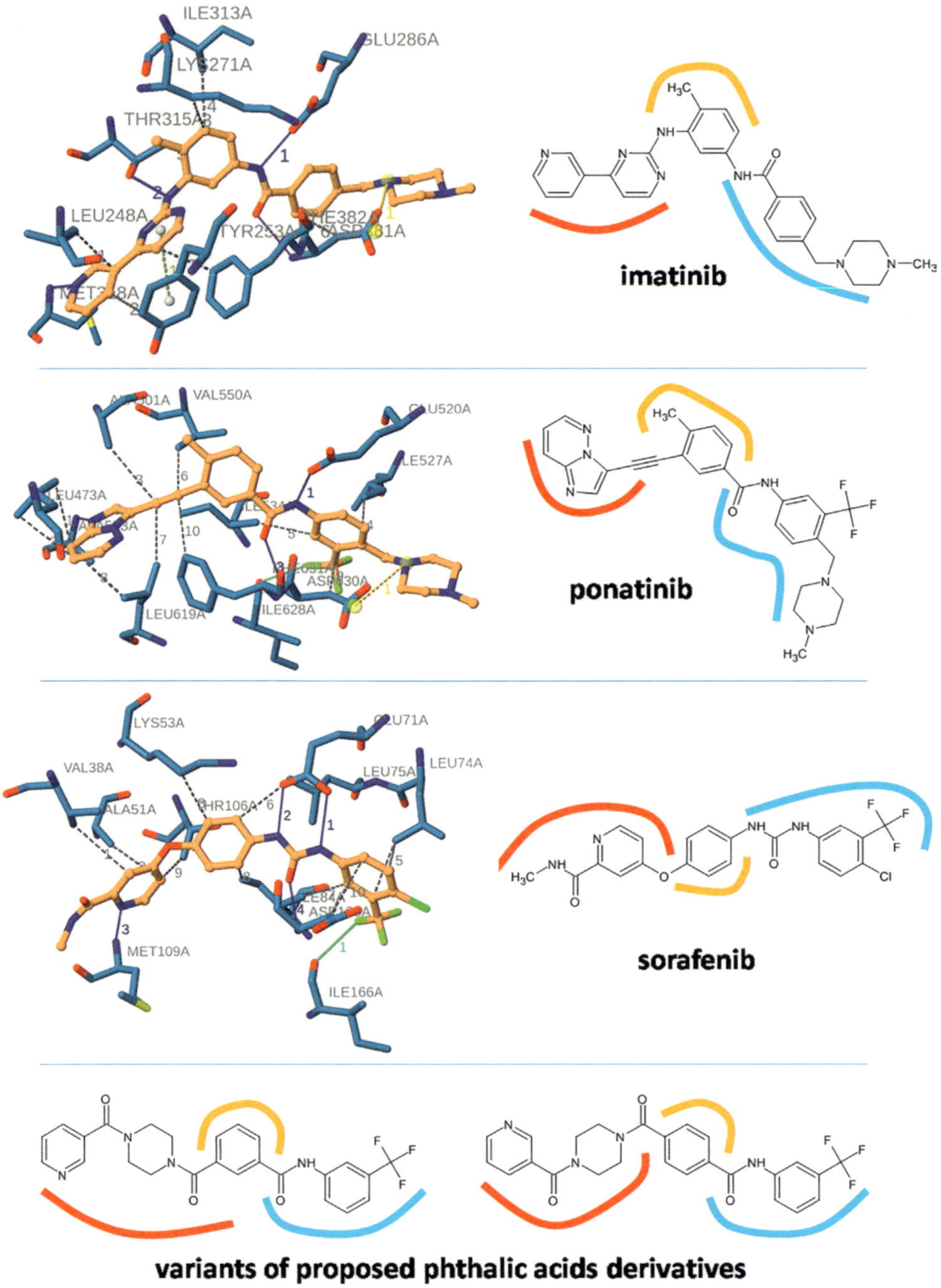

Figure 1.
Pharmacophore features of approved type 2 protein kinase inhibitors and proposed structures. Structural fragments that bind to different regions of binding site are highlighted with red (ATP pocket), blue (allosteric pocket), and orange (linker). Interactions were obtained by PLIP [47].

region. By varying the mutual arrangement of carbonyl groups, it could be possible to determine which linker is more suitable to be placed in a kinase's binding site.

On the basis of selected linkers, we have generated a library of novel chemical structures by introducing different amines into the carbonyl groups of phthalic acids

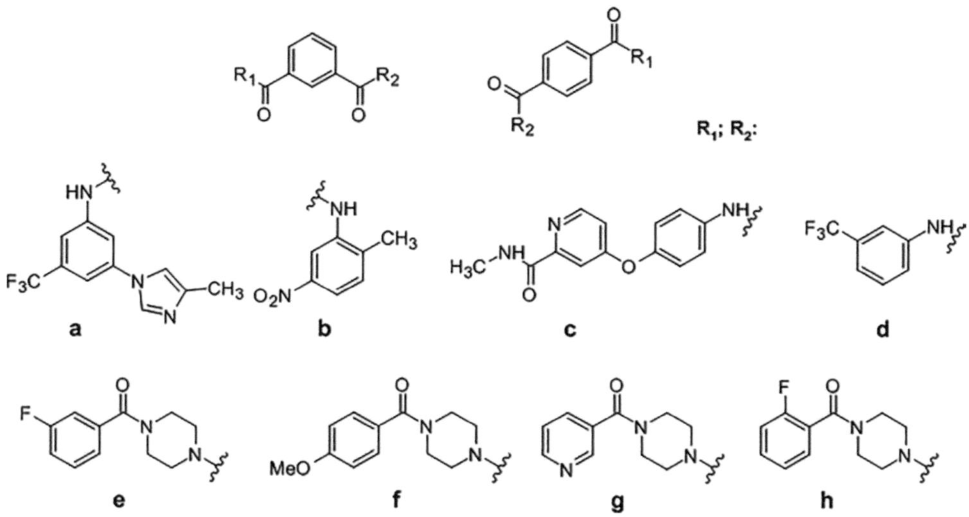

	a	b	c	d	e	f	g	h
a	IT	IT		IT	IT	IT	T	IT
b								
c	IT	IT	I	IT				
d				I	IT	IT	T	IT

Figure 2.
The generation scheme of studied phthalic acids derivatives. Letters a-h represent amine substituents. Letters I, T, and IT represent what type of linker was used for a structure: Isophthalic, terephthalic, or both.

to study their potential anti-kinase activity by molecular modeling and molecular docking. A total of 28 unique chemical structures are generated (**Figure 2**). As substituents at carbonyl groups of phthalic linkers, we have used structural fragments of known inhibitors: 3-trifluoroaniline (nilotinib, ponatinib, and sorafenib), 4-(4-aminophenoxy)-N-methylpyridine-2-carboxamide (sorafenib), and other amines convenient in terms of commercial availability and possibility of further derivatization.

2.2 Docking

For molecular docking experiments, 3D structures of studied phthalic acid derivatives are generated using the Cactus service [48]. For docking studies, we have used open-source software AutoDock Vina [49] as Qvina 2.1 [50] modification.

The 3D structures of 33 cancer-relevant protein kinases are used as docking receptors. Their structures are obtained from the database of experimental X-ray data The Protein Data Bank (PDB) [51]. Most of the receptors are protein kinases of different families. Two receptors are poly (ADP-ribose)-polymerases as this protein class is also used for targeted cancer therapy [52] (**Table 1**).

Docking of the constructed ligands and receptors is performed using “each to each” scheme. Coordinates of active centers for Qvina are generated based on a visual assessment of the location of native ligands from PDB complexes with an increase of approximately 10–30% in each dimension. The Qvina search exhaustiveness parameter is set to 24. The preparation of receptors and ligands for the docking has been performed using Chimera 1.13.1 [54].

	PDB code	Protein family	Original (native) ligand	Ligand binding type
1	1r0p	c-Met	Alkaloid K-252a	1
2	2bfy	Aurora-B	Hesperadin	1
3	2hyy	Abl	Imatinib	2
4	2in6	Wee1	PD311839	1/2
5	2pl0	Lck	Imatinib	2
6	2vrz	Aurora-B	ZM447439	1/2
7	3bbt	ErbB4 (Her4)	Lapatinib	1/2
8	3cs9	Abl	Nilotinib	2
9	3gcs	P38-Map	Sorafenib	2
10	3hng	Vegfr1	N-(4-chlorophenyl)-2-[(pyridin-4-ylmethyl)amino] benzamide	2
11	3og7	Braf V600E	PLX4032	2
12	3 pp0	ErbB2 (Her2)	2-{2-[4-({5-chloro-6-[3-(trifluoromethyl)phenoxy] pyridin-3-yl}amino)-5H-pyrrolo[3,2-d]pyrimidin-5-yl]ethoxy}ethanol	2
13	3qrj	Abl T315I	Rebastinib (DCC-2036)	2
14	3wze	Vegfr2 (kdr)	Sorafenib	2
15	3zbf	Ros1	Crizotinib	1
16	4ag8	Vegfr2	Axitinib (AG-013736)	2
17	4asd	Vegfr2	Sorafenib	2
18	4at3	Trkb	CPD5N	1/2
19	4b8m	Aurora-B	VX-680	1/2
20	4c2w	Aurora-B	ATP	1
21	4dce	Alk	(3S)-N-(4-methylbenzyl)-1-{2-[(3,4,5-trimethoxyphenyl)amino]pyrimidin-4-yl} piperidine-3-carboxamide	1/2
22	4g5p	Egfr T790M	BIBW2992	1
23	4lmn	Mek1	GDC0973 + ATP	—
24	4tvj*	Parp2	Olaparib	—
25	5ew9	Aurora A	MK-5108	1
26	5hi2	Braf	Sorafenib	2
27	5kup	Btk	6-{tert}-butyl-8-fluoranil-2-[3-(hydroxymethyl)-4-[1-methyl-6-oxidanylidene-5-(pyrimidin-4-ylamino) pyridin-3-yl]pyridin-2-yl]phthalazine-1-one	
28	5kvt	Trka	Entrectinib	1
29	5toz**	Jak3	PF-06651600	1
30	5y5u	Syk	4-[(1-methylindazol-5-yl)amino]-2-(4-oxidanylpiperidin-1-yl)-8H-pyrido[4,3-d] pyrimidin-5-one	1

31	6kzd	Trkc	3-[2-[6-(4-aminofenyl)imidazo[1,2-a]pyrazin-3-yl] ethynyl]-2-methyl-{N}-[3-(4-methylpiperazin −1-yl)-5-propan-2-yl-phenyl]benzamide	2
32	6nec	Ret	Nintedanib	1
33	7kk4*	Parp1	Olaparib	—

**A receptor is poly (ADP-ribose)-polymerase.*
***A ligand is a covalent inhibitor – it binds to the receptor by forming a chemical bond [53].*

Table 1.
Receptors used for the docking studies.

2.3 Molecular dynamics

After the docking step, the most promising protein-ligand complexes have been subjected to molecular dynamics simulation for more accurate binding affinity estimation. The complexes for the simulation are selected based on the obtained docking scores. The open-source GROMACS 2019.1 [55] software is used to conduct molecular dynamics experiments. The standard molecular dynamics protocol includes a minimization step, two 200 ps equilibration steps, and a final 2 ns simulation. The resulting molecular dynamics trajectory is used to estimate the binding energy, which is performed in three ways. All ligands are parameterized by Acpype [56]. Complete md-protocol is described in previous work [37].

The first two calculation methods include the implementations of the molecular mechanics Poisson-Boltzmann surface area (MM-PBSA) and molecular mechanics-generalized Born surface area (MM-GBSA) [57]. These methods are widely used to estimate inhibitory activity for protein-ligand complexes. Their main advantage is the relatively high accuracy of obtained results along with a simpler system setup procedure if compared to the thermodynamic integration or free energy perturbation methods [58]. A relatively short simulation time is chosen based on the published evidence that the accuracy of the MM-PBSA/MM-GBSA protocols is in many cases are independent of simulation time, and in some experiments a short simulation time is preferable [59].

In our case, the MM-PBSA/MM-GBSA binding energy calculation has been carried out using two kinds of softwares: g_mmpbsa [60] and gmx_MMPBSA [61]. The main difference between these programs, apart from the technical implementation, is that g_mmpbsa only calculates the Poisson-Boltzmann surface area (PBSA) variant, whereas gmx_MMPBSA allows to also using the generalized Born surface area (GBSA) and also provides entropy change estimation.

The third approach used provides the estimation of the binding affinity of the studied phthalic derivatives applying the RF-Score-VS (Random Forest-based scoring function for Virtual Screening) machine learning algorithm [39]. This algorithm uses a "set of decision trees" model trained on a large set of active and inactive docking poses. The main purpose of RF-Score-VS is to refine the estimation of docking results. In training procedure for this model, a set of deliberately inactive ligands are used aimed to increase the probability of distinguish real "hits" between the structures with the highest scores. This is what makes RF-Score-VS different from many other rescoring protocols, including RF-Score v3 [62] from the same authors, which are focused on more accurate numerical estimation of binding energy for known ligands. According to the published data [39], the RF-Score-VS model is significantly superior to the AutoDock Vina scoring function in terms of the probability of finding a real inhibitor. In our study, we have extended the scope of RF-Score-VS uses by applying it not to the obtained docking pose, but to the frames of the resulting molecular dynamics trajectory. In our opinion, this approach can be more accurate as it takes into account time-dependent changes of the protein-ligand complex reflected by the simulation. At the same time, the computing expenses remain acceptable.

In all three methods, we did not use the full 2-ns-long trajectory of the complex, but every 20th frame skipping first 200 ps of the production run.

3. Results and discussion

After docking stage, we obtained 924 complexes of the studied structures along with the corresponding docking scores representing binding energy estimation. In order to study any binding patterns, the resulting docking poses were filtered based on their binding energy. Docking scores better or equal to −11.5 kcal/mol were used as a threshold for filtering. This threshold was chosen based on our previous experience. After filtering, we obtained 133 docking poses out of 924 that showed such a high binding energy. We investigated then the distribution of filtered docking poses by linker type (isophthalic or terephthalic), by the most frequent amine fragments and by receptor type.

Out of 133 poses with high docking scores, 101 poses corresponded to the structures containing an isophthalic linker; therefore, 22 poses belonged to the structures having terephthalic linker. This ratio remained virtually unchanged when the filtration threshold was increased: 63/12 for the threshold of 12.0 kcal/mol and better, 30/8 at 12.5 kcal/mol, and 20/5 at 13.0 kcal/mol.

The distribution of amine substituents in high-scoring docking poses is shown in **Figure 3**. Amines containing 3-trifluoromethylaniline are the most frequent.

The most frequent receptors in protein-ligand complexes with a score of −11.5 kcal/mol and better are trkc kinase (PDB: 6kzd), abl family (PDB: 3cs9, 2hyy), and vegfr family (PDB: 3hng, 3wze, 4asd), as shown in **Figure 4**. It is important to note that all of these receptors are essentially protein kinases being in inactive conformation accepting type 2 ligands, which indirectly confirms the correctness of the chosen approach to the design of studied phthalic derivatives.

The obtained docking results indicate that the isophthalic linker, together with the attached 3-trifluoromethylaniline, might be a promising structural fragment in terms of its ability to bind to protein kinases as type 2 inhibitor.

At the second stage, we selected 25 complexes of the studied structures that were obtained during the docking step to refine ligand binding energies using molecular dynamics methods. The complexes for molecular dynamics simulation were chosen based on their docking score and to get a certain degree of diversity in chosen linkers and receptors. Out of 25 complexes, seven had terephthalic linker and 18 contained isophthalic linker.

After conducting a 2-ns simulation for each complex, we calculated the binding energy via processing the obtained trajectory frames using three methods: MM-PBSA (g_mmpbsa), MM-GBSA (gmx_mmpbsa), and rescoring with the RF-Score-VS scoring function. The last is based on a machine learning model (**Table 2**).

It was of particular interest for us to compare the results obtained by three methods of binding energy estimation. In our case, the values of electrostatic and van der Waals interactions obtained by g_mmpbsa (MM-PBSA) and gmx_mmpbsa

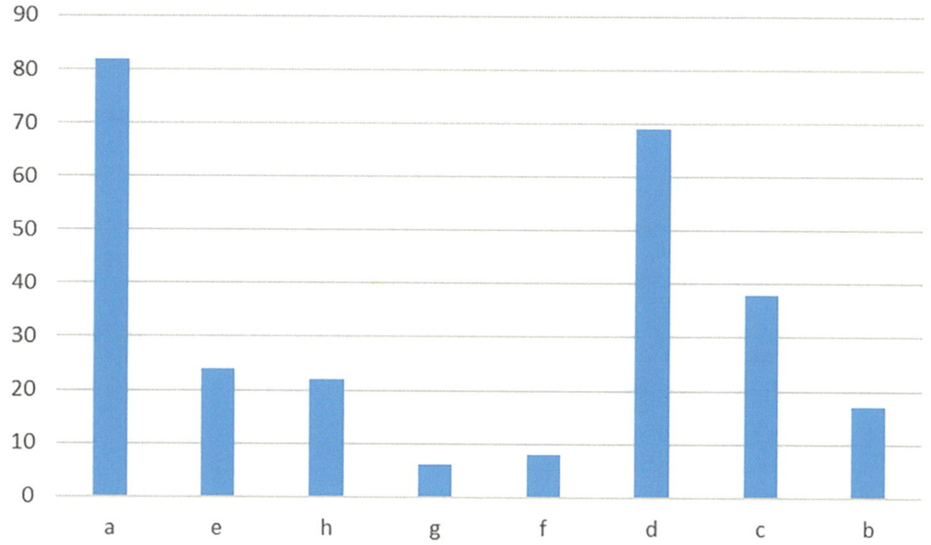

Figure 3.
Frequency of different amine fragments appearing in docking poses with a score of −11.5 kcal/Mol and better.

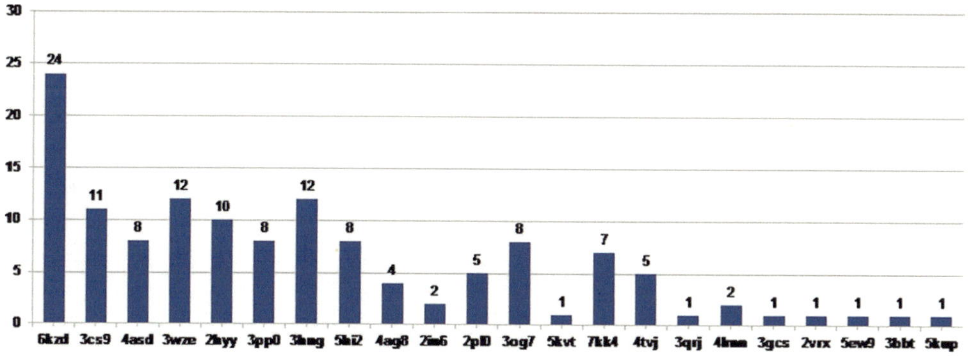

Figure 4.
Distribution of docking poses with a score of −11.5 kcal/Mol and better by receptor type.

(MM-GBSA) are in strict linear correlation with each other (**Figure 5**), which indicates that the methods for calculating the molecular-mechanical component of binding energy in these two tools are uniform.

When taking into account the solvation component, the correlation between this two methods decreases but remains high with the correlation coefficient R^2 = 0.76. The decrease in correlation can be naturally explained by the differences in the estimation of the solvation component of binding energy applying the Poisson-Boltzmann surface area and the generalized Born surface area. When the entropic component of gmx_mmpbsa is added, the correlation coefficient decreases slightly more but remains high (R^2 = 0.66). Thus, in general, both used programs show similar results for the same complexes.

We also compared the results obtained from MM-PBSA/MM-GBSA calculations with those of RF-Score-VS machine learning algorithm. The RF-Score-VS values moderately correlated both with the g_mmpbsa (R^2 = 0.50) and gmx_mmgbsa (R^2 = 0.51)

pdb	Linker	Amines		gmx_mmpbsa, kcal/mol				RF-score	g_mmpbsa, kJ/mol		
				v.d.w.	electr.	entr.	total		v.d.w.	electr.	total
3wze	iso	c	a	−71,1	−26,2	9,9	−48,8	**6,5**	−297,4	−54,7	−150,5
6kzd	iso	a	f	−65,8	−40,7	17,8	−31,4	6,3	−275,3	−85,14	−95,59
6kzd	iso	a	h	−62,7	−4,4	16,2	−31,4	6,1	−262,3	−9205	−111,5
3cs9	iso	a	h	−72,6	−13,5	6	−53,3	**6,3**	−303,5	−28,01	−144,9
6kzd	iso	a	e	−70,1	−20	9,9	−45,6	6,2	−293,4	−41,89	−137,9
6kzd	tere	a	h	−69,6	−19	18,7	−38,8	6,2	−291,3	−39,37	−141,1
6kzd	iso	d	h	−59,3	−2,4	13,3	−34,5	6,0	−248	−5111	−123,5
6kzd	tere	d	e	−58,1	−29,8	8,6	−39,3	6,0	−243,1	−62,39	−128,4
6kzd	iso	d	e	−48,5	−30,7	14,4	−21,5	6,0	−202,8	−64,39	−76,8
3 pp0	iso	d	e	−55,6	−9,1	7,7	−34,1	6,0	−232,6	−19,04	−96,72
6kzd	tere	a	e	−63,8	−5,5	15,2	−27,4	6,2	−266,7	−11,69	−125,9
5hi2	iso	d	h	−57,4	−27,4	7	−46,6	6,1	−240,2	−57,45	−118,9
3cs9	iso	d	h	−62,6	−14	13,2	−41	6,2	−262	−29,21	−128,6
3wze	iso	a	h	−74	−30,8	7,4	−64	**6,5**	−309,6	−64,57	−157
3wze	tere	d	e	−51,9	−30,3	8	−34,7	6,0	−217	−63,19	−85,65
6kzd	tere	a	g	−69,2	−12,5	9,9	−40,8	**6,4**	−289,5	−26,05	−134,3
3cs9	iso	c	a	−77,1	−37,1	9,1	−47,9	**6,3**	−322,3	−77,15	−144,4
3cs9	iso	d	f	−68	−21,6	13,8	−46	6,1	−284,4	−43,96	−141,8
6kzd	tere	a	f	−69,8	−22,4	14,2	−37	6,2	−291,8	−46,92	−149
4asd	iso	c	a	−79,9	−33,8	10,1	−53,6	**6,5**	−334,2	−70,75	−155,3
3hng	iso	a	d	−64,9	−22,6	16	−36,8	**6,3**	−271,3	−47,31	−119,6
3 pp0	tere	d	h	−50,8	−15,6	11,5	−26,7	6,0	−212,6	−32,59	−86,55

4ag8	iso	c	a	−76,4	−34,4	9,3	−53,5	**6,5**	−319,5	−71,87	−150,8
4ag8	iso	a	d	−65,4	−23,2	11,2	−44	6,2	−273,6	−49,12	−138,8
4ag8	iso	d	f	−65,2	−33,1	7,7	−58	6,2	−272,9	−69,09	−148,4
Reference ligands											
2hyy	imatinib			−67,4	−20,1	5,3	−50,5	6,2	−282,1	−42,4	−154,7
3cs9	nilotinib			−72,8	−28,1	6,1	−56,1	6,6	−304,6	−57,8	−183,1
3 pp0	original			−71	−19,5	12,7	−50,2	6,5	−297,1	−41,1	−143,6
6kzd	original			−82,6	−37,7	8,2	−61	6,4	−345,5	−66,2	−206,9

Table 2.
Calculated binding affinities of studied and reference structures to their receptors.

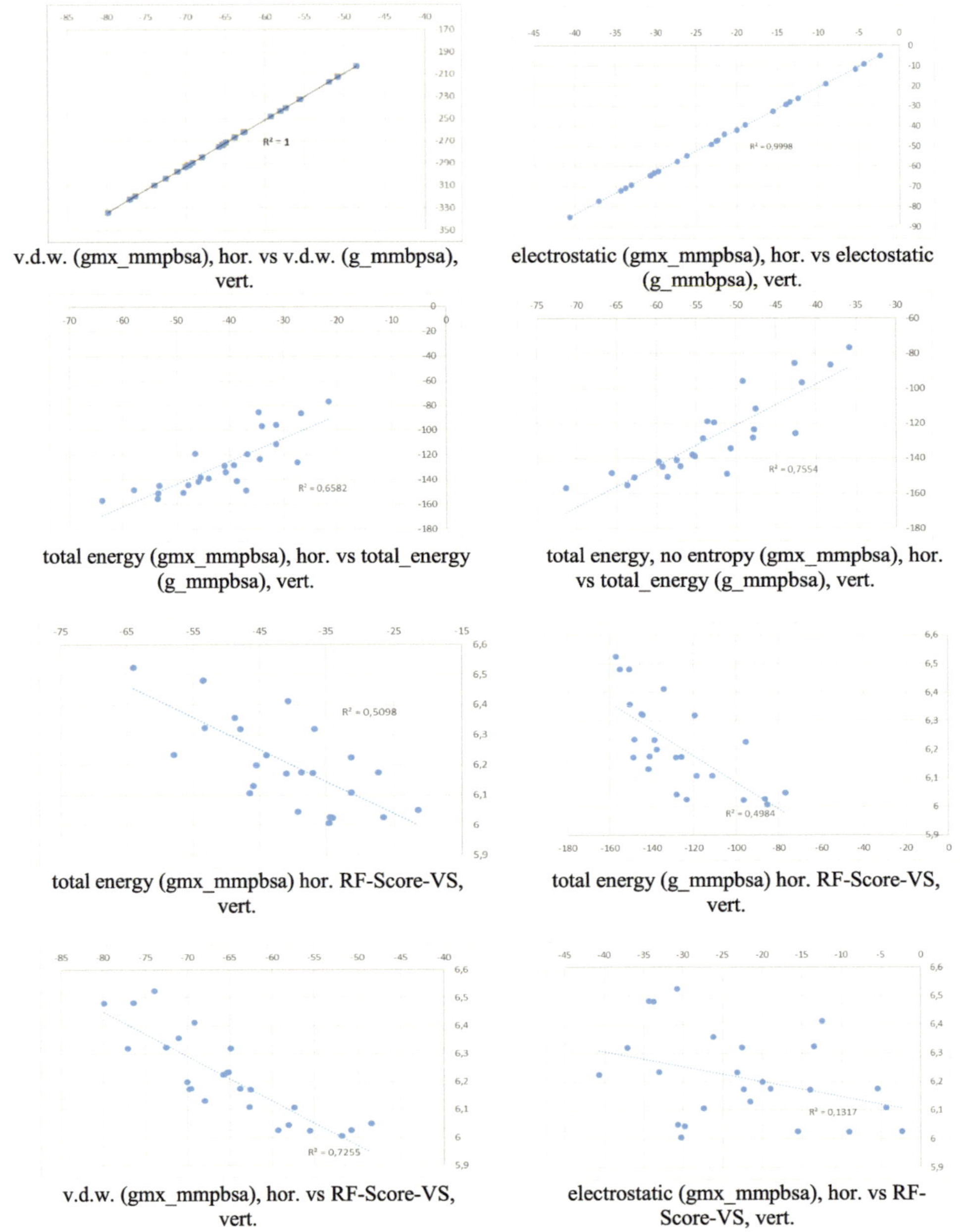

Figure 5.
Correlations between binding affinities obtained by different approaches.

final scores. It is noteworthy that the correlation between RF-Score-VS values and the van der Waals component of MM-PBSA/MM-GBSA binding energy is quite high (R^2 = 0.73) and extremely low for the electrostatic component (R^2 = 0.13).

All used methods for binding energy estimation are known to be more efficient for the relative ranking of potential inhibitors than for the precise calculation of absolute binding energy. Therefore, we have used known inhibitors as reference structures. In most cases, the studied phthalic derivatives showed worse binding energy scores compared to known inhibitors. The latter, in turn, were characterized by relatively high binding energy scores regardless the applied method for the calculation. Among the known inhibitors, the highest RF-Score-VS scores were observed for nilotinib (PDB id: 3cs9). Extremely high MM-PBSA/MM-GBSA energies were obtained for the native ligand of trkc kinase complex (PDB id: 6kzd). In the case of abl-protein kinase, nilotinib, being a second-generation inhibitor, showed higher estimated activity compared to the first-generation drug imatinib.

Among the studied phthalic acid derivatives, two structures can be distinguished which showed high binding energy scores calculated by all three methods. Both of these structures are isophthalic acid derivatives and contain a 5-imidazolyl-3-trifluoraniline fragment of nilotinib. The second carboxyl group in these structures is modified by 4-(4-aminophenoxy)-N-methylpicolinamide **a** (sorafenib fragment) and (2-fluorophenyl) (piperidin-1-yl) methanone **h**, respectively. If compared to known inhibitors, high *in silico* inhibitory activity of these structures was observed for vegfr receptors (pdb ids: 4asd, 4ag8, 3wze) and, to a slightly lesser extent, for abl (3cs9).

Several complexes of two aforementioned structures have been subjected to hydrogen bonds analysis. For the frames of the molecular dynamics trajectory, hydrogen bonds are searched using GROMACS hbond module. The frames with the highest number of hydrogen bonds have been visualized. Visualization shows that this structures bind to the active center similar to known type 2 inhibitors: the 3-trifluoromethylaniline fragment occupies the allosteric pocket and the isophthalic acid fragment plays a linker role. In both cases, the allosteric amide bond forms two hydrogen bonds with amino acid residues of asparagine and glutamine, which is typical for type 2 inhibitors (**Figure 6**). Regarding the ATP binding site, our analysis shows that the carbonyl group of phenyl (piperazin-1-yl) methanone may be involved in hydrogen bonding. In the case when 4-(4-aminophenoxy)-N-methylpicolinamide is located in this region, hydrogen bonds can be formed by oxygen atoms of phenolic and carbonyl groups. Hydrogen bonds of the non-allosteric amide bond of the phthalic linker have not been detected.

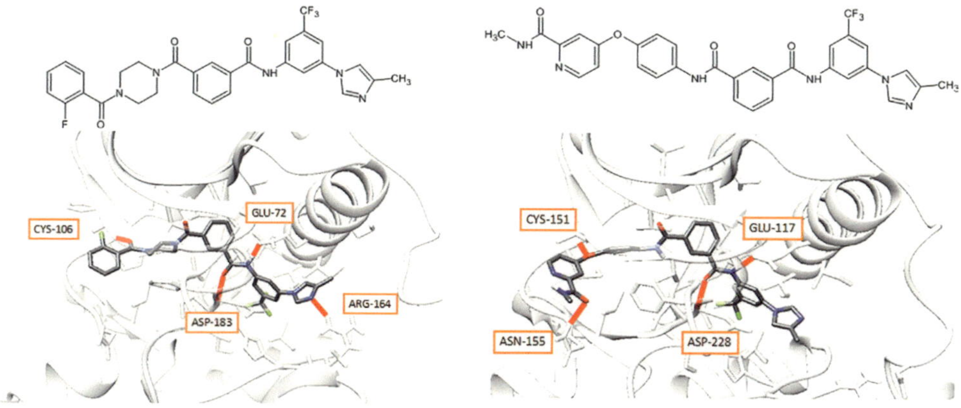

Figure 6.
Structure of most promising structures and the visualization of their binding to receptors. The binding of 3-(4-(2-fluorobenzoyl)piperazine-1-carbonyl)-N-(3-(4-methyl-1H-imidazol-1-yl)-5-(trifluoromethyl)phenyl) benzamide to vegfr is shown on the left (PDB id: 3wze, h-bonds: Cys-106, Asp-183, Glu-72, Arg-164. The binding of N1-(3-(4-methyl-1H-imidazol-1-yl)-5-(trifluoromethyl)phenyl)-N3-(4-((2-(methylcarbamoyl)pyridin-4-yl)oxy)phenyl) isophthalamide to vegfr is shown on the right (PDB id: 4asd, h-bonds: Cys-151, Asn-155, Asp-228, Glu-117).

4. Conclusions

In this study, 28 unique chemical structures of new derivatives of terephthalic and isophthalic acids have been studied. These structures are designed in such a way as to give the structures a significant pharmacophore similarity with known type 2 protein kinase inhibitors. Three-dimensional structures of 33 protein kinases associated with cancer have been used as docking receptors. At the same time, most of the receptors represent protein kinases of different families. The obtained docking parameters, the binding energy of MM-PBSA/MM-GBSA, and the affinity of RF-Score-VS suggest that the isophthalic linker together with the attached 3-trifluoromethylaniline may be a promising structural fragment in terms of its ability to bind to protein kinases as a type 2 inhibitor. In comparison with known inhibitors, high inhibitory activity of isophthalic structures in silico are observed for vegfr (pdb ids: 4asd, 4ag8, 3wze) receptors and to a somewhat lesser extent for abl (3cs9). If compared to known inhibitors, high in silico inhibitory activity of these structures was observed for vegfr receptors (pdb ids: 4asd, 4ag8, 3wze) and, to a slightly lesser extent, for abl (3cs9). At the same time, the use of terephthalic acid for this purpose is ineffective. The most promising structural fragment is 1-[3-(trifluoromethyl)phenyl]benzene-1,4-dicarboxamide. By introducing different substituents to the free amino group to this structure, the anti-kinase activity of the obtained chemical compounds can be expected.

Acknowledgements

This research was funded by the National Academy of Sciences of Belarus within the research project number 2.3.2.1 of State Program for Scientific Research "Chemical basis of life processes (bioorganic chemistry)."

Author details

Aliaksandr Faryna* and Elena Kalinichenko
Institute of Bioorganic Chemistry, National Academy of Sciences of Belarus, Minsk, Belarus

*Address all correspondence to: farina@iboch.by

References

[1] Kantarjian HM, Talpaz M. Imatinib mesylate: Clinical results in Philadelphia chromosome-positive leukemias. Seminars in Oncology. 2001;**28**(5 Suppl. 17):9-18

[2] Lyseng-Williamson K, Jarvis B. Imatinib. Drugs. 2001;**61**(12):1765-1776. DOI: 10.2165/00003495-200161120-00007

[3] Druker BJ, Tamura S, Buchdunger E, et al. Effects of a selective inhibitor of the Abl tyrosine kinase on the growth of Bcr-Abl positive cells. Nature Medicine. 1996;**2**(5):561-566. DOI: 10.1038/nm0596-561

[4] Witte ON, Dasgupta A, Baltimore D. Abelson murine leukaemia virus protein is phosphorylated in vitro to form phosphotyrosine. Nature. 1980;**283**(5750):826-831. DOI: 10.1038/283826a0

[5] Kantarjian H, O'Brien S, Jabbour E, et al. Improved survival in chronic myeloid leukemia since the introduction of imatinib therapy: A single-institution historical experience. Blood. 2012;**119**(9):1981-1987. DOI: 10.1182/blood-2011-08-358135

[6] Hochhaus A, Larson RA, Guilhot F, et al. Long-term outcomes of Imatinib treatment for chronic myeloid leukemia. The New England Journal of Medicine. 2017;**376**(10):917-927. DOI: 10.1056/NEJMoa1609324

[7] Roskoski R Jr. Properties of FDA-approved small molecule protein kinase inhibitors: A 2022 update. Pharmacological Research. 2022;**175**:106037. DOI: 10.1016/j.phrs.2021.106037

[8] Cohen P, Cross D, Jänne PA. Kinase drug discovery 20 years after imatinib: Progress and future directions. Nature Reviews. Drug Discovery. 2021;**20**(7):551-569. DOI: 10.1038/s41573-021-00195-4

[9] Ghosh S, Marrocco I, Yarden Y. Roles for receptor tyrosine kinases in tumor progression and implications for cancer treat-ment. Advances in Cancer Research. 2020;**147**:1-57. DOI: 10.1016/bs.acr.2020.04.002

[10] Kleczko EK, Heasley LE. Mechanisms of rapid cancer cell reprogramming initiated by targeted receptor tyrosine kinase inhibitors and inherent therapeutic vulnerabilities. Molecular Cancer. 2018;**17**(1):60. DOI: 10.1186/s12943-018-0816-y

[11] Lovly CM, Shaw AT. Molecular pathways: Resistance to kinase inhibitors and implications for therapeutic strategies. Clinical Cancer Research. 2014;**20**(9):2249-2256. DOI: 10.1158/1078-0432.CCR-13-1610

[12] Tartarone A, Lazzari C, Lerose R, et al. Mechanisms of resistance to EGFR tyrosine kinase inhibitors gefitinib/erlotinib and to ALK inhibitor crizotinib. Lung Cancer. 2013;**81**(3):328-336. DOI: 10.1016/j.lungcan.2013.05.020

[13] Lamontanara AJ, Gencer EB, Kuzyk O, Hantschel O. Mechanisms of resistance to BCR-ABL and other kinase inhibitors. Biochimica et Biophysica Acta. 2013;**1834**(7):1449-1459. DOI: 10.1016/j.bbapap.2012.12.009

[14] Dong RF, Zhu ML, Liu MM, et al. EGFR mutation mediates resistance to EGFR tyrosine kinase inhibitors in NSCLC: From molecular mechanisms to clinical research. Pharmacological Research. 2021;**167**:105583. DOI: 10.1016/j.phrs.2021.105583

[15] Daver N, Schlenk RF, Russell NH, Levis MJ. Targeting FLT3 mutations in AML: Review of current knowledge and evidence. Leukemia. 2019;**33**(2):299-312. DOI: 10.1038/s41375-018-0357-9

[16] Yu HA, Arcila ME, Hellmann MD, Kris MG, Ladanyi M, Riely GJ. Poor response to erlotinib in patients with tumors containing baseline EGFR T790M mutations found by routine clinical molecular testing. Annals of Oncology. 2014;**25**(2):423-428. DOI: 10.1093/annonc/mdt573

[17] Castellanos E, Feld E, Horn L. Driven by mutations: The predictive value of mutation subtype in EGFR-mutated non-small cell lung cancer. Journal of Thoracic Oncology. 2017;**12**(4):612-623. DOI: 10.1016/j.jtho.2016.12.014

[18] Roskoski R Jr. Targeting oncogenic Raf protein-serine/threonine kinases in human cancers. Pharmacological Research. 2018;**135**:239-258. DOI: 10.1016/j.phrs.2018.08.013

[19] Fletcher JA, Rubin BP. KIT mutations in GIST. Current Opinion in Genetics & Development. 2007;**17**(1):3-7. DOI:10.1016/j.gde.2006.12.010

[20] Broekman F, Giovannetti E, Peters GJ. Tyrosine kinase inhibitors: Multi-targeted or single-targeted? World Journal of Clinical Oncology. 2011;**2**(2):80-93. DOI: 10.5306/wjco.v2.i2.80

[21] Bayazeid O, Rahman T. Correlation analysis of target selectivity and side effects of fda-approved kinase inhibitors. Chemistry Select. 2021;**6**(30):7799-7814

[22] Casado P, Alcolea MP, Iorio F, et al. Phosphoproteomics data classify hematological cancer cell lines according to tumor type and sensitivity to kinase inhibitors. Genome Biology. 2013;**14**(4):R37. DOI: 10.1186/gb-2013-14-4-r37

[23] Chakraborty S, Lin YH, Leng X, et al. Activation of Jak2 in patients with blast crisis chronic myelogenous leukemia: Inhibition of Jak2 inactivates Lyn kinase. Blood Cancer Journal. 2013;**3**(9):e142. DOI: 10.1038/bcj.2013.41

[24] Gambacorti-Passerini C, Aroldi A, Cordani N, Piazza R. Chronic myeloid leukemia: Second-line drugs of choice. American Journal of Hematology. 2016;**91**(1):67-75. DOI: 10.1002/ajh.24247

[25] Saglio G, Kim DW, Issaragrisil S, et al. Nilotinib versus imatinib for newly diagnosed chronic myeloid leukemia. The New England Journal of Medicine. 2010;**362**(24):2251-2259. DOI: 10.1056/NEJMoa0912614

[26] Manley PW, Drueckes P, Fendrich G, et al. Extended kinase profile and properties of the protein kinase inhibitor nilotinib. Biochimica et Biophysica Acta 2010;1804(3):445-453. doi:10.1016/j.bbapap.2009.11.008

[27] Weisberg E, Manley P, Mestan J, Cowan-Jacob S, Ray A, Griffin JD. AMN107 (nilotinib): A novel and selective inhibitor of BCR-ABL. British Journal of Cancer. 2006;**94**(12):1765-1769. DOI: 10.1038/sj.bjc.6603170

[28] Zhou N, Xu Y, Liu X, et al. Combinatorial pharmacophore-based 3D-QSAR analysis and virtual screening of FGFR1 inhibitors. International Journal of Molecular Sciences. 2015;**16**(6):13407-13426. DOI: 10.3390/ijms160613407

[29] Sharma A, Thelma BK. Pharmacophore modeling and virtual screening in search of novel Bruton's tyrosine kinase inhibitors. Journal of

Molecular Modeling. 2019;**25**(7):179. DOI: 10.1007/s00894-019-4047-y

[30] Srivastava S, Mehta P, Sharma O, Sharma M, Malik R. Computationally guided identification of Akt-3, a serine/threonine kinase inhibitors: Insights from homology modelling, structure-based screening, molecular dynamics and quantum mechanical calculations. Journal of Biomolecular Structure & Dynamics. 2020;**38**(14):4179-4188. DOI: 10.1080/07391102.2019.1675536

[31] Hu Y, Zhou L, Zhu X, Dai D, Bao Y, Qiu Y. Pharmacophore modeling, multiple docking, and molecular dynamics studies on Wee1 kinase inhibitors. Journal of Biomolecular Structure & Dynamics. 2019;**37**(10):2703-2715. DOI: 10.1080/07391102.2018.1495576

[32] Li Y, Pu Y, Liu H, et al. Discovery of novel wee1 inhibitors via structure-based virtual screening and biological evaluation. Journal of Computer-Aided Molecular Design. 2018;**32**(9):901-915. DOI: 10.1007/s10822-018-0122-1

[33] Holderbach S, Adam L, Jayaram B, Wade RC, Mukherjee G. RASPD+: Fast protein-ligand binding free energy prediction using simplified physicochemical features. Frontiers in Molecular Biosciences. 2020;**7**:601065. DOI: 10.3389/fmolb.2020.601065

[34] Wang S, Liu D, Ding M, et al. SE-OnionNet: A convolution neural network for protein-ligand binding affinity prediction. Frontiers in Genetics. 2021;**11**:607824. DOI: 10.3389/fgene.2020.607824

[35] Macari G, Toti D, Pasquadibisceglie A, Polticelli F. Docking app RF: A state-of-the-art novel scoring function for molecular docking in a user-friendly Interface to auto dock Vina. International Journal of Molecular Sciences. 2020;**21**(24):9548. DOI: 10.3390/ijms21249548

[36] Ballester PJ, Mitchell JBA. Machine learning approach to predicting protein-ligand binding affinity with applications to molecular docking. Bioinformatics. 2010;**26**(9):1169-1175. DOI: 10.1093/bioinformatics/btq112

[37] Kalinichenko E, Faryna A, Bozhok T, Panibrat A. Synthesis, In vitro and In Silico anticancer activity of new 4-Methylbenzamide derivatives containing 2,6-substituted purines as potential protein kinases inhibitors. International Journal of Molecular Sciences. 2021;**22**(23):12738. DOI: 10.3390/ijms222312738

[38] Kalinichenko E, Faryna A, Kondrateva V, et al. Synthesis, biological activities and docking studies of novel 4-(Arylaminomethyl) benzamide derivatives as potential tyrosine kinase inhibitors. Molecules. 2019;**24**(19):3543. DOI: 10.3390/molecules24193543

[39] Wójcikowski M, Ballester PJ, Siedlecki P. Performance of machine-learning scoring functions in structure-based virtual screening. Scientific Reports. 2017;**7**:46710. DOI: 10.1038/srep46710

[40] Nagar B, Bornmann WG, Pellicena P, et al. Crystal structures of the kinase domain of c-Abl in complex with the small Mol-ecule inhibitors PD173955 and imatinib (STI-571). Cancer Research. 2002;**62**(15):4236-4243

[41] Roskoski R Jr. Classification of small molecule protein kinase inhibitors based upon the structures of their drug-enzyme complexes. Pharmacological Research. 2016;**103**:26-48. DOI: 10.1016/j.phrs.2015.10.021

[42] Vijayan R.S, He P, Modi V, et al. Conformational analysis of the DFG-out kinase motif and biochemical profiling of structurally validated type II inhibitors. Journal of Medicinal Chemistry 2015;58(1):466-479. doi:10.1021/jm501603h

[43] Wan PT, Garnett MJ, Roe SM, et al. Mechanism of activation of the RAF-ERK signaling pathway by oncogenic mutations of B-RAF. Cell. 2004;**116**(6):855-867. DOI: 10.1016/s0092-8674(04)00215-6

[44] Chan WW, Wise SC, Kaufman MD, et al. Conformational control inhibition of the BCR-ABL1 tyrosine kinase, including the gatekeeper T315I mutant, by the switch-control inhibitor DCC-2036. Cancer Cell. 2011;**19**(4):556-568. DOI: 10.1016/j.ccr.2011.03.003

[45] O'Hare T, Shakespeare WC, Zhu X, et al. AP24534, a pan-BCR-ABL inhibitor for chronic myeloid leukemia, potently inhibits the T315I mutant and overcomes mutation-based resistance. Cancer Cell. 2009;**16**(5):401-412. DOI: 10.1016/j.ccr.2009.09.028

[46] Suebsuwong C, Pinkas DM, Ray SS, et al. Activation loop targeting strategy for design of receptor-interacting protein kinase 2 (RIPK2) inhibitors. Bioorganic & Medicinal Chemistry Letters. 2018;**28**(4):577-583. DOI: 10.1016/j.bmcl.2018.01.044

[47] Adasme MF, Linnemann KL, Bolz SN, et al. PLIP 2021: Expanding the scope of the protein-ligand interaction profiler to DNA and RNA. Nucleic Acids Research. 2021;**49**(W1):W530-W534. DOI: 10.1093/nar/gkab294

[48] NCI Chemical Identifier Resolver. Available from: http://cactus.nci.nih.gov/chemical/structure [Accessed: December 13, 2021]

[49] Trott O, Olson AJ. AutoDock Vina: Improving the speed and accuracy of docking with a new scoring function, efficient optimization, and multithreading. Journal of Computational Chemistry. 2010;**31**(2):455-461. DOI: 10.1002/jcc.21334

[50] Alhossary A, Handoko SD, Mu Y, Kwoh CK. Fast, accurate, and reliable molecular docking with QuickVina 2. Bioinformatics. 2015;**31**(13):2214-2216. DOI: 10.1093/bioinformatics/btv082

[51] Berman HM, Westbrook J, Feng Z, et al. The protein data Bank. Nucleic Acids Research. 2000;**28**(1):235-242. DOI: 10.1093/nar/28.1.235

[52] Slade D. PARP and PARG inhibitors in cancer treatment. Genes & Development. 2020;**34**(5-6):360-394. DOI: 10.1101/gad.334516.119

[53] Abdeldayem A, Raouf YS, Constantinescu SN, Moriggl R, Gunning PT. Advances in covalent kinase inhibitors. Chemical Society Reviews. 2020;**49**(9):2617-2687. DOI: 10.1039/c9cs00720b

[54] Pettersen EF, Goddard TD, Huang CC, et al. UCSF chimera--a visualization system for exploratory research and analysis. Journal of Computational Chemistry. 2004;**25**(13):1605-1612. DOI: 10.1002/jcc.20084

[55] Van Der Spoel D, Lindahl E, Hess B, Groenhof G, Mark AE, Berendsen HJ. GROMACS: Fast, flexible, and free. Journal of Computational Chemistry. 2005;**26**(16):1701-1718. DOI: 10.1002/jcc.20291

[56] Sousa da Silva AW, Vranken WF. ACPYPE - AnteChamber PYthon parser interfacE. BMC Research Notes.

2012;**5**:367. DOI: 10.1186/1756-0500-5-367

[57] Kollman PA, Massova I, Reyes C, et al. Calculating structures and free energies of complex molecules: Combining molecular mechanics and continuum models. Accounts of Chemical Research. 2000;**33**(12):889-897. DOI: 10.1021/ar000033j

[58] Pu C, Yan G, Shi J, Li R. Assessing the performance of docking scoring function, FEP, MM-GBSA, and QM/MM-GBSA approaches on a series of PLK1 inhibitors. Medchemcomm. 2017;**8**(7):1452-1458. DOI: 10.1039/c7md00184c

[59] Genheden S, Ryde U. The MM/PBSA and MM/GBSA methods to estimate ligand-binding affinities. Expert Opinion in Drug Discovery. 2015;**10**(5):449-461. DOI: 10.1517/17460441.2015.1032936

[60] Kumari R, Kumar R. Open source drug discovery consortium, Lynn a. g_mmpbsa--a GROMACS tool for high-throughput MM-PBSA calculations. Journal of Chemical Information and Modeling. 2014;**54**(7):1951-1962. DOI: 10.1021/ci500020m

[61] Valdés-Tresanco MS, Valdés-Tresanco ME, Valiente PA, Moreno E. gmx_MMPBSA: A new tool to perform end-state free energy calculations with GROMACS. Journal of Chemical Theory and Computation. 2021;**17**(10):6281-6291. DOI: 10.1021/acs.jctc.1c00645

[62] Li H, Leung KS, Wong MH, Ballester PJ. Improving AutoDock Vina using random Forest: The growing accuracy of binding affinity prediction by the effective exploitation of larger data sets. Molecular Informatics. 2015;**34**(2-3):115-126. DOI: 10.1002/minf.201400132